To Candy & Roger,

· Know your options
· Listen to your inner voice
· Choose

Dette Jo Arnett

WHOLEISTIC
DENTISTRY

WHOLEISTIC DENTISTRY

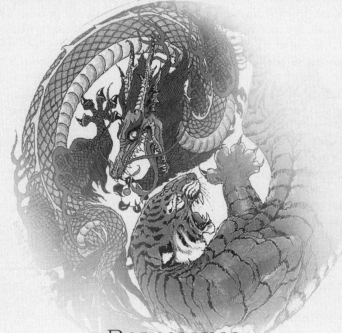

BALANCING
CONVENTIONAL DENTAL CARE
WITH
ANCIENT WISDOM

BETTE JO ARNETT

BEAVER'S
POND
PRESS

ISBN 10: 1-59298-430-4
ISBN 13: 978-1-59298-430-5

Library of Congress Catalog Number: 2011933597

Printed in the United States of America

First Printing: 2011

15 14 13 12 11   5 4 3 2 1

Cover and interior design by James Monroe Design, LLC.

Beaver's Pond Press
7104 Ohms Lane, Suite 101
Edina, MN 55439–2129
952-829-8818
www.BeaversPondPress.com

To order, visit www.BeaversPondBooks.com
or call 1-800-901-3480. Reseller discounts available.

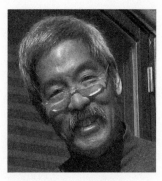

1948 – 2010

Dedicated to Ron King, DDS.

*You inspired me by your vision and bravery,
always encouraging your dental colleagues to know
their patients and empowering your patients
to know their options.*

CONTENTS

FOREWORD

Holistic medicine is widely accepted in the twenty-first century. Most medical professionals seem to understand that a malfunction of one body part impacts others. Further, most medical professionals accept that human physiology, chemistry, psychology, and spirituality are closely interrelated. Moreover, Eastern and Western healing techniques have merged. Acupuncture is now covered by most health insurers just like physical therapy, surgery, and prescription pharmaceuticals. So what happened to the dental profession?

Modern dentistry is on the cusp of a new era. Thanks to innovative dentists like the late Dr. Ronald King, DDS, a holistic approach has been increasingly integrated into dental practice. More important, holistic dentistry is becoming integrated with holistic medicine. After all, isn't the mouth—with its teeth, gums, and jaw—part of the whole body? That's the point of this book: Teeth and kidneys can impact one another, jaw and stress are related, gums and the chemistry of digestion influence one another.

In this book, Bette Jo Arnett addresses both the dental professional and the patient. To the dental professional she says, "The teeth and gums are not your only responsibility. Your patient is a whole person with a history and a multifaceted environment. Your patient may have an allergy that limits your treatment options. Your patient's body and soul influence physiological responses to your treatments. Your patient is complex." To the patient, Arnett says, "Know your options. Understand your whole body. Beware of unnecessary or inappropriate treatments. Dentists don't intend to harm you—sometimes they just don't understand all of you. Help them. Explain the whole you."

Arnett builds bridges between dentist and patient. The two desperately need to understand one another if holistic medicine and conventional care are to work properly. We must begin to build a common language of holistic dentistry that can lead to a common understanding. Communication theory asserts that "language is culture and culture is language." As Arnett teaches us a new language of holistic medicine, she starts to build a new culture in the dental office. This new culture is Arnett's vision and the centerpiece of her book.

Arnett's examples are meant to be generalized. The dental professional and the patient must learn the principles she teaches. When she tells us that some people are allergic to mercury in fillings while other patients show no negative reactions, we learn a principle: Be alert to potential allergies. When Arnett suggests that bridges and implants can cause negative reactions, she is not recommending against these procedures; she is simply pointing out that human beings are complex and often unpredictable organisms. Therefore patients should know all their options, including the option of doing nothing, before they make a decision. Further, patients should know that if they experience negative reactions, treatments can often be reversed. For example, dental bridges can be removed.

In sum, this book provides a grand vision of a new and more complex practice of dentistry that understands mind, body, and environment. Bette Jo Arnett is a visionary speaking to dental professionals and patients. I join Arnett in hoping for an additional audience that will find this book useful: the dental educator.

Fred M.B. Amram
Morse Alumni Distinguished Professor Emeritus of
Creativity and Communication

PREFACE

My stomach tightened with anger as I worked on my patient, a twenty-seven year old who wanted to get her teeth cleaned before she had a kidney transplant in two weeks. Six years earlier she had been diagnosed with lupus. The same year she had two dental bridges placed on her lower jaw. She had to struggle for several years with the auto-immune effects of Lupus. She came to the holistic dental office hoping to find answers to her illness.

When the nickel allergy was discovered, the damage to her kidneys was too great. The bridges in her mouth contained nickel. When, I thought, will my conventional colleagues ever understand? When a twenty-one year old has been diagnosed with an autoimmune illness, do you think, just maybe, someday these professionals will look for the connection of the illness to the dentistry they performed in the last year?

After she left, my anger turned to sadness. I thought about her the rest of the day and all the other patients I have seen in similar situations that my profession calls anecdotal. My sadness turned to despair. It felt hopeless. What can a few holistic dental professionals do to change a huge institution to transcend into another paradigm in health care? What can we say to bring awareness of the pain that might be prevented by insightful dental care?

To the readers

In the last seventeen years I have seen impressive healing with homeopathy for my family and clients. As well, my dental patients, many of whom are healers or clients of alternative medicine, share stories of results from these therapies.

My faith in alternative medicine comes from my father. I am the daughter of a dowser. My school years were spent defending my father and his great gift with my public school teachers. Their science could not comprehend or explain how he could find water, deep in the Earth, with a stick. As I watched him connect with a power greater than words could explain, I came to know there is great mystery. It is not important to always know how things work, but to trust that they do. This faith is the foundation for my work with energy medicine and homeopathy.

From my education in dentistry, homeopathy, and coaching, it is my desire to share words to inspire others on their journeys, words that help others to focus on their paths, and words to motivate people to make choices that will achieve balance and harmony.

PART
I

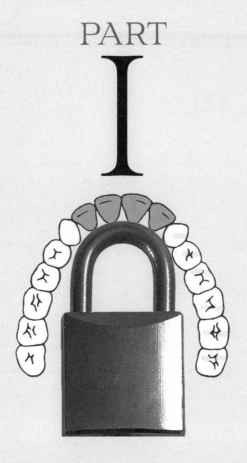

ARE YOU BETTER OFF WITHOUT
YOUR BRIDGE?

ONE

Introduction

We shall never cease from exploration
And at the end of all our exploring
Will be to arrive where we started
And know the place for the very first time

T. S. Elliot (Dacher, 2006, p. 62)

As it has advanced, the profession of dentistry has helped millions of patients experience dental work in the most pain-free way and with the best restorative techniques. American dentistry is the best I have seen in patients from all parts of the world. However, when establishing and updating protocols, dentistry has not taken into account knowledge from other disciplines, like Chinese and Tibetan medicines, which are based on the meridian theory and balance of the individual person (Dorjee, 2005). These Eastern medical models have been used for thousands of years to treat individual suffering, yet their benefits to modern dentistry have remained largely unexplored.

My experience in holistic dentistry and homeopathy prompts me to ask questions of my profession. Are we

1

professionals placing materials in and performing procedures on patients that prevent the balance necessary to
maintain health? Are dental treatments creating a bioburden of toxins that promote or develop chronic illness?
In other words, are the materials we place in a patient's
mouth, such as fluoride, gold, silver, and tooth-colored fillings, compatible with that patient's biochemistry? Or is it
possible that some patients have allergies to these materials? Could symptoms that indicate a chronic illness, like
lupus or other autoimmune diseases, come from an imbalance in the body as a result of dental work?

In addition, can dental materials or dental procedures,
such as root canals and extractions of infected teeth, over-
whelm the body's ability to eliminate toxins effectively?
Does a dental bridge, which crosses the midline of the palate on the upper front teeth, lock the bones of the palate
so that they cannot move? Will a locked palate prevent the
body from proper structural movement and then create
symptoms of disease for the patient? I will address all of
these questions in this book from the viewpoint of a holistic health practitioner.

The majority of American dentists support the American Dental Association (ADA) protocols for practice. Fewer
believe that the protocols that use mercury/silver fillings
(known as dental amalgam,) or procedures such as dental
bridges, root canals, fluoride treatments, or treatments for
cavitations (pockets of infection within the bone), might
cause harm to some patients. These dentists believe in dental care as it relates to the whole person and give patients
different choices about their care. They are called holistic
dentists. They recognize the potential of dental work to
affect the overall general health of an individual, and point
to the number of patients with adverse affects linked to
dentistry (HDA, 2008).

From my experience with holistic techniques and

homeopathy, I have observed that patients could benefit from the integration of the Eastern philosophy of traditional Chinese/Tibetan medicine into conventional dental practices. How can this be done, however, when the training standards and protocols for practice are set by the ADA?

All dentists in the United States must abide by ADA protocols or they will not be allowed to practice dentistry. As a result, some dentists who use Eastern concepts of medicine have been driven from practice. The most famous of them is Hall Huggins, a Colorado dentist who lost his license in 1994 after continued investigation by the licensing board (Radford, 2003). He believed in and used concepts relating to balancing the body chemistry and was testing patients for sensitivity to materials.

The ADA resists incorporating an understanding of holistic Eastern philosophy and methods into training and protocols. As evidence, the ADA has approved using silver fillings to restore teeth, even though they contain 50% mercury, a neurotoxin, since its inception in 1859. This toxin is known to affect the whole body as it galvanizes from dental fillings (Haley, 2001). Yet, holistic dentists must be careful when discussing this galvanism with patients. They risk losing their licenses to practice if they recommend an option that might contradict a protocol set by the dental association (Sullivan, 2004).

In this book, I examine the benefits of integrating the two philosophies and what it will take to make integration possible. How would integrating conventional dentistry with traditional Chinese and/or Tibetan medicines benefit dental patients? What are the factors preventing the ADA from integrating these holistic principles? I believe that economics, politics, and a lacking in understanding of the benefits of traditional Chinese/Tibetan medicine prevent this integration. As I make the case for this, I explore the positions of the ADA, holistic dentists, the Eastern

3

philosophies of Chinese and Tibetan medicines, and the benefits of integrating the two philosophies. I hope to show how integration might take place through coaching techniques and invention, producing a model that has the potential to make both patients and dentistry whole.

In the course of my exploration, I evaluate accounts of holistic dentists regarding claims of harm from their websites, scientific studies, books about dentistry, and my personal experience in the dental profession with holistic techniques. The ADA website and my training as a hygienist and former educator of dental hygiene provide the foundation of expectations of the conventional dental protocols. As a homeopath, I draw from books about alternative medicine and my private consultations with clients to show how the energy in the individual is disrupted by conventional dentistry.

The second chapter defines some terminology and discusses the concepts of traditional Chinese and Tibetan medicines. The third chapter discusses the philosophy of conventional dentistry and how it contrasts with holistic-based dentistry, as well as how a holistic dental practitioner uses the concepts of traditional Chinese and Tibetan medicines. I address the factors that prevent integration of these holistic concepts into United States dentistry in chapter four, and chapter five explores the possibility of integration of holistic concepts into dentistry in the future. Chapter six details the knowledge that patients will need to generate questions they must ask to obtain holistic care from their conventional dentist. In the last chapter, I draw conclusions about why the integration has not already taken place and what needs to happen before the profession of dentistry moves forward to include holistic concepts in their protocols for dental professionals.

TWO

DEFINING THE TWO WORLD VIEWS

Choose a middle road between too much and too little . . . just as both overeating and under eating will lead to poor health, even a noble cause, when carried too far becomes harmful. A middle path will take both action and its results into account.

MIRIAM CAMERON (CAMERON, 2001, P. 59)

Conventional Dentistry

By "conventional dentistry" I mean the dental practices in the United States of America governed by the state dental boards in accordance with the standards set by the ADA (ADA, 2010). In 1859, a small group of twenty-six like-minded dentists supporting the use of silver fillings formed the ADA (Wynbrandt, 1998). This organization established ethical guidelines for practicing dentistry, as well as positions on materials that could be used and how they were to be used.

Today, the ADA sets standards for the education of dental professionals and auxiliaries. Anyone performing dental procedures in the United States is governed by the ADA, as are all schools, public and private, that educate dental professionals.

Each state board of dentistry licenses dentists working in its state. Additionally, each state board abides by the standards and guidelines set by the ADA. About 70 percent of all U.S. dentists belong to the organization and pay a membership fee (ADA, 2010). The remaining dentists do not belong, but must abide by the guidelines of the ADA in order to practice dentistry in the United States. A dentist's reason for not belonging to the professional dental organization might range from not needing to in order to practice dentistry to having differences in philosophy.

The Holistic Dental Professional

Holistic dentists are also governed by the guidelines set by the ADA. They view their role differently from that of the conventional dentist, however. Holistic dentists understand the body as a whole, with every part relating to every other part. Even more significantly, they understand the materials and procedures used to restore teeth as having effects on the rest of the body (HDA, 2008).

Both conventional and holistic dental practitioners acknowledge that a patient's dental health can affect his or her body. For example, they agree that a patient's poor brushing and flossing habits can cause gum disease and that bacteria from the mouth can cause infections in other parts of the body, such as the heart. Habits like cigarette smoking can also promote poor oral health. But this is where the similarity ends between the two. As noted earlier, the holistic dentist goes further, acknowledging that a patient's mouth is a reflection of her or his entire body. As a result, a holistic dentist will regard problems in the mouth as potential signs of greater problems in the body. That is to say, the holistic dentist may suspect that the patient's dental work may be contributing to ill health, or her dental work may be contributing to her overall ill health.

For example, to a holistic dentist, unexplained bone loss around the teeth may indicate bone loss throughout the other hard tissues of the body in the form of osteoporosis. The conventional dentist, however, may regard the bone loss as caused by poor dental home-care techniques, lack of home care, or destructive behaviors, such as smoking. While these factors *can* contribute to bone loss, the holistically minded dentist or hygienist will consider that bone loss is often a symptom of an underlying cause on the mental, emotional, or physical plane.

Holistic dentistry is based on the principles of traditional Chinese and Tibetan medicines. Practitioners believe that the parts of the body are interconnected through meridians or channels that also run through the teeth (Dorjee, 2005). Therefore, when one tooth is being restored, an entire meridian of the body is affected. For example, a dental restoration on the lower right first premolar would be situated on an energy channel that runs through that tooth. This particular channel also runs through the pancreas, liver, pylorus, and stomach. It also affects thoracic vertebrae numbers eleven and twelve, as well as the first lumbar vertebrae (King, 2010).

According to the traditional approach, organs, muscle groups, nerves and other anatomical structures along the meridian would be affected by that dental restoration. The ADA, however, points to the lack of evidence, viewing this approach to medicine as anecdotal and pseudoscientific.

And this response is typical; the ADA does not support the ancient practice of traditional Chinese or Tibetan medicines as they relates to dental care.

Energy Medicine Philosophy

Many disciplines make up the general field of energy medicine, and homeopathy is one of them. So are traditional Chinese medicine and Tibetan medicine. Hands-on healing, Reiki, and acupuncture are also energy medicine. For convenience's sake, I will use the frameworks provided by traditional Chinese medicine and Tibetan medicine to explain core concepts in energy medicine, the most critical of which is the principle of individualized treatment, which is the basis for my argument and comes from the philosophy of these ancient disciplines.

Traditional Chinese medicine, a healthcare system that has been in existence for thousands of years, is based on the Daoist–Confucianist idea of holism. According to holism, the body is seen as a reflection of the world. In other words, the body is a microcosm of the macrocosm. As a consequence, what happens in the world affects the individual person. And just as individuals relate to one another in the world and affect one another, the body parts relate to one another and affect one another. In essence, individual people and an individual person's body parts are all interdependent (Beinfield & Korngolld, 1995).

In essence, traditional Chinese and Tibetan medicines contend that there is a correspondence between the greater world and the inner world of the person. Therefore, a relationship exists between the teeth and the body.

The holistic dentist also sees the mouth as a reflection of what is happening in the person's body. What can this look like? If a person has bone loss around his teeth, he may have an imbalance in blood pH, which reveals the blood's acidity or alkalinity. In humans, blood *must* remain at 7.4 pH. If the blood pH is 7.3 or lower, the body will display acidosis, or have too much acid. When this happens, the body will attempt to restore balance by pulling calcium from the bones. If the person suffers from acidosis often enough, a dentist will likely see bone loss around the teeth.

Because holistic dental professionals recognize that a patient's mouth and body reflect the health of one another, they also believe that materials used to restore the teeth can affect the rest of the body. This means that a dental procedure such as drilling can affect the entire person. As well, the interaction of the patient and the practitioner affects the patient on the mind, body, and spiritual levels (Dorjee, 2005, p. 129). Also, a material used in filling the teeth can create a blockage of energy flowing through the body, and this block may result in the formation of toxins.

While the ancient principle of holism holds that the parts of the body reflect the greater whole, it highlights another critical relationship: the relationship between the body, mind, and spirit. According to traditional holism, the body is a place where the spirit and the mind live and animate what we know as a human being (Dorjee, 2005). And the consequences of this for holistic dentistry are significant.

Holistic dental practitioners believe that each patient's personal-care habits, as well as their mental outlooks toward dental procedures or life in general, can alter his or her body chemistry, which in turn ultimately affects both dental and overall health (Dorjee, 2005). When a patient is going through a stressful time in her personal life, such as pregnancy, puberty, or chronic illness, or losing a job, her teeth and mouth may be affected. Thus, a person's physical wellbeing may mirror the wellbeing of her spiritual, emotional, and mental life.

Even with this brief discussion, it is clear that traditional Chinese and Tibetan medicines differ from Western medicine practiced in the United States. The latter is based on reductionism, or the breaking apart of what's complex into its simpler parts. In fact, this is the core of Western medical philosophy. Accordingly, the body is seen as a machine, with parts that need to be evaluated, replaced, or repaired. Western medical philosophy recognizes that the parts of the body interrelate to keep it running, but the body is seen rather like a car, where fuel is necessary to make the car run or pistons are needed to perpetuate motion. There is little acknowledgement that a soul or spirit animates the body or that energy meridians connect parts of the body, including the teeth (Beinfield, & Korngolld, 1995).

Traditional Tibetan Medicine

Traditional Tibetan medicine is similar to traditional Chinese medicine, but it is more spiritually based. It is one of the world's oldest medical systems and is grounded on the idea that, while all things are interrelated, there is a continual push and pull between opposite forces. There is never a truly permanent form of anything, but rather an ebb and flow in all things at all times. Instead of producing an antagonism, this process of push and pull creates a positive relationship or a harmony (Dorjee, 2005).

Harmony is a compatibility in opinion or action or parts that creates a pleasing combination in a whole. Harmony creates a balance. A famous Tibetan picture provides a perfect example of this harmony: It is an image of an elephant with several animals balancing on its back, one on top of the other. This picture represents the interrelationship of all things and how they can live in harmony to achieve a positive end or benefit to all (Cameron, 2001). Yet, any harmonious balance can be disrupted. Imbalances can occur when we do not understand how things are interrelated.

The Tibetans believe that all illness starts in the mind. It results from some kind of imbalance and is revealed by the expression of one of three poisons: greed, jealousy, or closed mindedness. Traditional Tibetan medicine tries to restore balance by prescribing herbs or changes in diet, lifestyle, and behavior. In order to restore balance, a practitioner must first understand the person's underlying nature and the distribution of energy known as humours (Horowtitz, 2007).

Within this healing framework, practitioners assess an individual's nature in terms of three humours: *loong, tripa,* and *badkan.* These humours represent energies of air, fire, earth, and water and are always in the body. *Loong,* or air energy, coincides with desire, greed, and attachment. *Tripa,* or fire energy, coincides with anger, hatred, and fear. *Badkan,* or earth, is the energy of closed mindedness (Dorjee, 2005). All three energies are present in everyone and keeping them equally balanced is ideal; however, most humans have a predominant energy or constitution.

Each element has a positive quality. Earth energy is about being responsible and standing on our own. It is about consistency and faith and being grounded. Water is about moving with ease through life and our relationships. It is about joy and contentment in being alive. It is innate and not dependent on external circumstances. Fire represents the creativity of the mind and the digestive heat of the body. It is about warmth and developing wisdom and discrimination. Change and movement is represented by air and allows everything to be connected to see things from all different angles. It is the essential energy of existence or chi. Space accommodates all the other elements and makes

11

room for them and life to happen so that, whatever problems or discomforts are encountered, they can be handled with ease (Rinpoche, 2002).

The concept of humours can be used by holistic practitioners to help understand a patient's susceptibility to cavities or gum disease. Knowing a person's nature or constitution helps to guide a dental patient to a healthy diet and lifestyle.

The energies of the five elements affect us deeply and can be in or out of balance depending on what we do, eat, think about, or participate in with our family or society. The key in traditional Tibetan medicine is to learn which energies are out of balance and what is needed to rebalance them in order to achieve harmony.

Holistic Practitioners

The holistic dental practitioner takes into consideration that the patient has an individual nature and will often refer the patient to other practitioners skilled in energy concepts. These professionals will then recommend particular diets and behaviors that will rebalance the elements, given that different foods, actions, and even professions reflect the different elements and can be called up to ease imbalances. Unless specifically trained in Tibetan medicine, a dentist or hygienist may not be qualified to prescribe the needed changes, but knowledge of the concept of individuality will help them refer dental patients to alternative complimentary practitioners.

The alternative dental practitioner, like the homeopath or the naturopath, addresses symptoms to reveal the underlying causes of a patient's ill health or dental health, and will respond accordingly. To understand how an alternative dental practitioner might assess a patient's symptoms, consider an example. Imagine a holistic dentist with a twenty-something-year-old patient suffering from gum recession. An unusual condition for a young person, gum recession happens when the gums become diminished, leaving the roots of the teeth exposed.

To fully understand the patient's situation, the holistic dentist would first rule out that the recession was caused by the patient's bite or home care. Then he or she would refer the patient for a medical exam to determine if a chronic illness, like diabetes, might be the cause. Lastly, if no other cause is apparent, the dentist might refer the patient to a naturopath to address the pH balance of the patient's body. The naturopath would address all symptoms and prescribe changes to halt the gum recession.

Science in Dentistry

The ADA uses science as a measurement to include or exclude a treatment or a process involved in the care of a patient. Furthermore, the dental profession uses the rational method of science when setting protocols (ADA, 2010). The guidelines are based on the conventional Western medicine philosophy that draws on the thought of Rene Déscartes and Sir Isaac Newton.

The Cartesian–Newtonian model is based on a material, objective reality that can be measured and quantified. It separates the mind from the body, because the working of the mind cannot be measured or verified by the scientific methods set out in the Cartesian model. Most branches of Western medicine today, however, deal primarily with the body's anatomy and physiology; the mind is the object of study for the fields of psychiatry and psychology. As noted earlier, this approach views the human body as a machine, and its complex parts are broken down into smaller parts to be measured and quantified (Beinfield & Korngolld, 1995).

Scientific studies that essentially depend on the Cartesian-Newtonian model are also used to establish guidelines for practicing dentistry. For example, some of the materials used both historically and currently to restore teeth, such as dental amalgam, gold, porcelain, fluoride, and so forth, may have been subjected to tests on groups of people, like dental amalgam. The ADA has a Center for Evidence Based Dentistry that allows a dental professional to access a database of studies done on materials and dental care topics. This center helps dentists establish practices based on conclusions drawn by researchers regarding product safety for use in the dental office (ADA, 2010).

An Example of the Scientific Method in Dental Hygiene, an Auxiliary Dental Profession

One can see an example of this rational method in the way that dental hygiene students are taught to care for dental patients. Dental hygienist students learn to clean teeth and instruct patients in the proper methods of caring for their teeth. That is, they learn how to clean away soft and hard deposits from the teeth, take x-rays, give fluoride treatments, and educate patients about brushing and flossing the teeth. The method used to teach them is called the process of care (Mueller-Joseph, 1995).

In 1989, the American Dental Hygienist's Association Counsel on Education (part of the ADA) decided there was a need for a comprehensive plan for training dental hygienists. The intent was also to develop a theoretical framework for the practice of dental hygiene; up until that time, dental hygienists had been trained in technical skills through rote learning and intuition (Mueller-Joseph, 1995, p. 4). This proposed plan was developed and the standards are now followed by all dental hygiene schools in the United States. The goal of the training is to teach students how to develop and perform the technical skills, critical-thinking skills, and judgment needed to make decisions about the care of a dental patient.

In this process we see the influence of Rene Déscartes' *Rules for the Direction of the Mind*. Indeed, Descartes' rules are the historical basis for the scientific method. One of the main components is the breaking down of a complex problem into smaller and smaller parts in order to understand that problem. Déscartes also stresses the importance of fully understanding the smallest part before moving on to figure out the next-smallest part (Griffith, 1997).

How is this method evident in the process of care? The training of dental hygienists teaches students a method to assess the status of the patient and to predict any potential problems. This process of care method breaks down large problems, namely patient treatment, into smaller components, and adopting the method involves a progression from simple to complex thinking, and culminates in a critical evaluation of what each individual dental patient needs. The components of the process of care include: assessment, dental hygiene diagnosis, planning, implementation, and evaluation of success (Mueller-Joseph, 1995). These stepwise components mark the progression that student hygienists go through when aiming to understand and meet a patient's needs. According to the method, working with a patient using this progression is the ideal way for hygienists to determine the best care plans for their patients.

In the assessment stage, the student hygienist is taught

to collect subjective and objective data. The subjective data includes general information about the patient and his perceptions, feelings, and ideas about his dental and general health. An example of subjective information would be this: "I have cold sensitivity on the lower right side of my mouth." The student follows up with questions about how long the patient has had the condition and if it is a recurring problem in the patient's past history.

The student follows this subjective data assessment with an objective assessment of the condition of the patient's mouth. This is an actual visual exam of the area the patient is complaining about, although the hygienist looks at everything in the mouth. The student will note any irregularity in the teeth or gums and identify the exact area causing the sensitivity, adding this to other objective information required to fulfill the requirements of and move forward in the process of care.

After the observation, the student makes a diagnosis of the problem. Given our example of the patient complaining of pain when eating or drinking something cold, the student, upon examination and depending on what she saw during the exam, might diagnose that the gum tissue has receded on the first lower right molar, leaving the tooth exposed and susceptible to cold.

In the next step of the process of care, the student progresses to planning and decides what needs to be done to correct the problem. This could involve desensitizing the spot on the tooth with a topical preparation to give the patient relief.

The next step—implementation—involves cleaning deposits from the area or, in our example, the application of a desensitizer to the area with the tools needed to apply it. The dental hygiene student will prepare all the tools before starting the procedure.

Finally, the student documents in the patient's chart

all that was done. When the patient returns at a later date, the hygienist will evaluate if the procedure worked. By properly recording what she did, the dental professional is able to make an accurate assessment of completion and, if called for, design a new plan to bring desired results. If the plan needs revision, the same process is used for a new plan: assessment, diagnosis, planning, implementation, and evaluation.

This process is used for every part of the duties a dental hygienist performs on a patient. The process is always the same, whether it is applied to evaluating a complaint from the patient or an observation of the hygienist while performing her duties.

The process of care is a detailed progression that involves collecting and reflecting on basic information, giving the hygienist the ability to develop a way to think and act. This training is done systematically, helping the student to learn a method and to deliver care with a reliable and predictable outcome. The ideal is that hygienists consistently find what is best for each patient.

Comments on the process of care

The process of care that dental hygienists learn is an example of how dental training uses the scientific method. As it stands, however, it is not holistic. This process is not necessarily based on the idea that the health of a person's mouth reflects the health of that person's body, and vice versa. A holistic dental hygienist follows the steps outlined in the process of care. She would treat a patient complaining of cold sensitivity in the same manner as a conventional hygienist, but she would go a step further, looking for a cause of the recession that presented the symptom of cold sensitivity in the first place.

The additional step in a holistic office would be to do an enzyme test to see if the recession of the gums is progressing and may result in additional sensitivity at a future date. One such test called the BANA (benzoyl-DL-arginine-napthylamide) test detects the presence of an enzyme found in three anaerobic bacteria that are associated with risk for gum disease (Oratec, 2010). It can be used to determine if the patient is at risk for future bone loss and sensitivity, as well as for a patient presenting with bleeding, pocketing, wear, or tooth erosion. It is comparable to the use of an x-ray to diagnose dental decay. By using the BANA test, one can discover pathology, which may lead to a deeper cause of interference in the localized site of the tooth and impact the patient's overall health. It is important to note that *any* dentist, conventional or holistic, could use this test.

A positive BANA is an opportunity for the dental professional and the patient to address causes for ill health. Once the practitioner determines the cause of the symptoms, she can determine if dentistry, inadequate home care, or general health problems have contributed. She can then recommend treatment. Furthermore, this test makes the patient aware of the risk of future gum problems. This approach determines and addresses both cause and symptom, and is superior to simply treating the symptom by prescribing better home care or shorter time between cleaning visits. The goal is to find the cause of the symptom, not to just suppress the symptom.

The holistic hygienist can use this test for any adult and to assess patients with one of the following indicators: recession 1+ mm, pockets 4+ mm, inflammation of the gums, bleeding, wear, or erosion. When recession or attrition are present, the practitioner will discuss options, such as returning for a structural/functional evaluation. If the results are positive, the practitioner might request that the patient return for a wellness consultation to evaluate diet, lifestyle, and medical history, of the option for referral to a medical doctor or alternative practitioners for treatment. The patient can take results from the BANA test to another holistic practitioner they see for care, or the patient might choose to do nothing.

If the patient wants to discover the cause of the sensitivity, the holistic dentist or hygienist can counsel him on holistic philosophy and how the sensitivity is an indicator of a deeper health concern. Such counseling would require that the practitioner take a detailed account of the patient's health history from childhood to the present, including a detailed account of diet, lifestyle, therapies, and the results that the patient has or has not tried. If no obvious conclusions result from the discussion, the holistic practitioner can refer the patient to other conventional and alternative practitioners.

The conventional approach to caring for dental patients is based on rational scientific protocols, while an individualized plan for discovering the cause of dental complaints is used by the holistic practitioner. The holistic dentist and hygienist follow the Eastern philosophy of recognizing the mouth as a reflection of the body. This may lead the patient to discover the underlying causes that have surfaced as symptoms in the patient's mouth.

Controversial Topics in Dentistry

Conventional and holistic dental practitioners view several topics in dentistry from different vantage points. They include the safety of root canal therapy, the use of fluoride in doses higher than the one part per million in the water supply, bridges that cross the midline of the palate, cavitations from extractions, periodontal disease, and dental materials, particularly silver fillings that contain mercury. In what follows, I discuss the silver filling controversy in some detail to establish an argument for the need to integrate Eastern concepts into dentistry. It is important to note that each of the other controversies can show how dental patients can benefit from the Eastern concept of individuality, however. Before I raise my concerns about silver fillings, I address each of these topics briefly, so that the reader does not assume that my concern is just about mercury in dental fillings.

Root Canals

Meining's book is about the research done on root-canalled extracted teeth by Weston Price, a dentist and nutritionist in the early 1900s. Holistic dentists believe that Price was correct when he concluded that bacteria in teeth are much like cancer cells that can metastasize to other parts of the body. Price conducted research over a twenty-five-year period along with a team of sixty researchers. He conducted his most famous experiment on a tooth extracted from a woman with crippling arthritis. Dr. Price pulled a root-canalled tooth, suspecting it to be the source of her suffering. He then placed the tooth under the skin of a rabbit. In two days the rabbit showed signs of crippling. Ten days after the tooth was imbedded under its skin, the rabbit died. Price went on to experiment further and discovered that whatever disease the patient had, the rabbits would develop it when he placed the extracted root-canalled teeth under their skin. The ADA and conventional dentists do not accept Price's theory, which is called focal infection and hypothesizes that infection can travel from the teeth to the body.

J. Craig Baumgartner states in an article regarding root-canalled teeth, "Endodontically treated or root canalled teeth alone does not cause bacteremia or systemic disease." This position is based on research done on guinea pigs in 1939. The researcher concluded that removal of the source of the infection by doing a root canal on the infected tooth eliminates any further infection (2002, p. 63). This finding became the basis for root canal treatment done today and is accepted as the standard by the ADA.

Baumgartner states that Dr. Price's research in the 1930s was poorly designed and is now outdated. However, the research done in 1939, only nine years later, is accepted as the standard for the millions of root canals dental patients experience every year. In *Root Canal Cover-up*, George Meinig states that Percy Howe and John Buckley waged the fight against the focal infection theory. Howe had injected streptococcus bacteria taken from a normal infection free mouth and injected it into rabbits. "None of the animals became sick or died" (p. 116). Buckley could not see how root canalled teeth which appeared to be free from infection could possibly create infection in the studies conducted by Price. Furthermore, some of the patients who had root-canalled teeth removed did not improve (p. 116).

The holistic practitioner contends that the conventional dental community ignores the fact that a dead tooth contains anaerobic bacteria that can live without oxygen in the microscopic tubules of the dentin of the tooth, and that it is impossible to sterilize all the tubules to prevent further infection. Price's research showed that bacteria become virulent and more dangerous because they were able to mutate and adapt to conditions (Meinig, 1998, p. 116). Price sterilized extracted teeth before implanting them into the animals. Even then, sterilization was unable to kill all of the bacteria, as evidenced when the same disease the patient had appeared in the rabbits.

Meinig maintains that antibiotics are unable to reach all the bacteria hiding in the dentinal tubules because the blood flow and nerve endings have been removed during the root canal procedure (p. 117). Researchers D. A. McGowan and J. M. Hardie validated Price's research in 1974. They showed in studies on rabbits that dental bacteria can be transferred to the heart, creating infective endocarditis. Today, it is routine to premedicate with antibiotics before dental treatment to prevent an infection from occurring in patients who have health concerns, like mitral valve prolapse or recent joint replacement. This is confirmation of the focal infection theory. However, the ADA stands by the belief that root canals do not cause any harm to patients.

Fluoride Controversy

Fluoride is used to prevent tooth decay in children and adults in the dental office and in prescription toothpaste for at-home use. Studies show that fluoride prevents decay in children and adults (Griffin, Regnier, Griffin, & Huntley, p. 410). Fluoride used in the dental office is in the form of gels, foams, or varnishes. It is placed on the teeth and releases the fluoride over minutes or hours. Fluoride paste is also available in prescription form for use at home. Patients are evaluated for their risk for tooth decay to determine which method would benefit them the most.

In addition, fluoride is in the water supply and is available in over-the-counter toothpastes. Since the early 1970s, the state of Minnesota has added fluoride to the drinking water at one part per million. Holistic-minded dental professionals agree that many studies show that fluoride prevents tooth decay. They question, however, is how much fluoride is safe to ingest and how much comes from multiple sources available from food, water, and dental products. Over-the-counter toothpaste can contain 1,000 to 1,500 parts per million. In-office fluoride treatments and varnishes contain 1,000 to 22,000 parts per million. If one part per million is considered safe in drinking water, what are the effects of many thousands of parts per million on a daily basis (CDC, 2010)?

Holistic practitioners are concerned for the overall health of the individual and cite studies that show adverse effects of fluoride on the thyroid and brain (Trabelsi, Guermazi, & Zeghai, 2001, p. 165). Since thyroid hormones are needed for the proper growth of the nervous systems and for brain development, this may have serious consequences. Some countries contain high levels of fluoride in their natural drinking water. Their population shows enlargement of the thyroid and a reduction of thyroxin in the blood. Studies done on pregnant and lactating mice show their babies have decreased body weight and brain proteins fourteen days after birth (p. 165).

Most every dentist and their auxiliaries can identify white spots, known as fluorosis, on some patients' teeth. This indicates too much fluoride. The holistic practitioner wants to know the answer to this question: If we see the effects on the patient's teeth, what is the effect on the rest of the body?

Cavitations Controversy

In 1915, dentist G. V. Black labeled bone necrosis or dead tissue of the jaw as chronic osteitis (Levy, 2010). Today they are called cavitations or NICOs, neuralgia-inducing cavitational osteo-necrosis. When a person has this condition, her jaw exhibits hollowed-out areas or pockets of dead tissue without any inflammation, bleeding, or fluid visible from the mouth. These areas are in extraction sites. Although they appear to be healed from the surface, when reopened surgically, they reveal necrotic tissue. Patients with this condition may experience unexplained pain or other health symptoms, like Parkinson's disease (Levy, 2010). Black described how to treat these areas by surgically removing the dead tissue, but his findings never became a part of modern dentistry.

Conventional dentists do not concur on how to diagnose cavitations because they are not always evident on a dental x-ray. Holistic dentists use symptoms of pain in extraction sites or electrical devices that measure bone density as a method of diagnosis. Diagnosis is elusive sometimes, but holistic dentists recommend protocols for treatment to prevent cavitations from occurring (Levy, 2010). Holistic dentists perform or request an oral surgeon to remove the periodontal ligament when a tooth is extracted. A motorized drill is used to grind out the ligament and remove some healthy bone.

Teeth are usually extracted when there is disease. Holistic dentists feel leaving the periodontal ligament of a diseased tooth prevents healthy bone from forming in the healing process. Then the site heals over the dead cells of the ligament, resulting in holes or cavitations that may appear months or years later.

Bridges Crossing the Midline

Conventional dentists place bridges crossing the midline of the patient's mouth every day. Little is written about this topic, but the holistic practitioner sees it as a potential problem for some patients. In chapter six, I will describe my personal experience to demonstrate the need for caution when placing bridges on the upper jaw.

These dental controversies, although I have described them only briefly, show there are aspects of dentistry that may harm dental patients. Those interested in a holistic approach to dentistry will want to explore these issues in more detail, since they are of concern for any individual when receiving or delivering dental care. I've chosen to discuss the dental amalgam and dental materials controversy in more detail because of the wealth of information available on the subject, as well as the urgency of the issue.

THREE

CONVENTIONAL DENTISTRY VS. HOLISTIC DENTISTRY

Whatever darkness we are unable to face within ourselves will manifest on the outside . . . this inevitably leads to the projection of our own inner problem onto some other person, group or nation . . .
whilst we sit back and proclaim our inner purity and goodness.

CARL JUNG (DORJEE, 2005, P. 141)

Conventional dentistry and holistic dentistry differ. The conventional dentist is driven by rational, mathematical, and scientific logic, activities of the left side of the brain. While holistic dentists are steered by the left-brain training they received in dental school, they also incorporate right-brain thinking, using intuition, instinct, emotions, and artistry. The conventional dentist has been shaped by strict ideals established by the ADA, which constructs them

27

into codes of ethics and positions about what is to be said and done when treating patients. The holistic dental professional, on the other hand, integrates mind-body-spirit concepts that guide his or her actions. Specifically, they recognize that patients respond uniquely on physically, mentally, and emotionally levels, and that their responses affect their dental and overall health. Along the way, each dentist, conventional or holistic, has developed approaches to their work and outlooks about how things should work when treating dental patients.

In this chapter, I discuss the philosophy of conventional dentistry, the practices of which are governed by the ADA, by focusing on the ADA position about filling materials. I then contrast this to the position of the Holistic Dental Association (HDA) and their concern that certain conventional dental practices and protocols actually harm dental patients' overall health. I use the controversial issue of dental amalgam, as well as the dental materials commonly used to restore teeth, as examples of how the two groups differ.

Dental Amalgam Position of the ADA

The ADA reports on their website that dental amalgam is safe and effective as a filling material. Amalgam fillings contain a combination of mercury, silver, copper, tin, and zinc. Dentists forming the ADA supported using dental amalgam fillings, even though there was controversy about the safety of fillings containing mercury. The research that the association accepts as valid allows them to conclude the following: There is no reason not to use amalgam to restore teeth.

The Food and Drug Administration, National Institute

of Dental Research, United States Public Health Service, National Multiple Sclerosis Society, and Consumers Union (publisher of *Consumer Reports*) all agree dental amalgam is safe to use. In August 2009, the FDA classified dental amalgam as Class II, which means moderate risk, rather than Class III, which means potentially hazardous. Amalgams do not require proof of safety or any warning to the public. Additionally, the FDA does not require any notice that dental amalgam contains mercury.

The ADA concurs with these other agencies; it maintains that when mercury is mixed with the other components that make up the amalgam filling, stable compounds result. In this way it is similar to hydrogen. When alone, hydrogen can be explosive, but it becomes stable when mixed with oxygen, forming water. While only trace amounts of metallic mercury remain in amalgam fillings, the governing body of dentists is convinced that small amounts of mercury vapor escaping from amalgams do not affect humans adversely.

Amalgam is an easy material to work with and place as a restoration. The area in need of filling, for example, does not have to be kept dry to successfully place the filling. This is ideal when working on unwilling children in the dental chair. Amalgam is also very cost effective and takes less time to place than other filling material.

For the past 160 years, dental professionals have placed thousands of amalgams daily. Studies show there is no correlation between patient complaints of illness and exposure to dental amalgam (ADA, 2010). If there was a problem with exposure to dental amalgams, dental staff would be the most likely to suffer. They are in constant contact in the dental office with fumes from initial placement or replacement of amalgam fillings. Yet, data shows that dental personnel have good or better health than the general population (ADA, 2010).

The ADA claims that testimonials of improved health after amalgam removal are not balanced with reports of patients who did not have improvement after amalgam removal. Therefore, they feel it is not a valid claim to have a concern for placing dental amalgam. Perhaps as a result of the ADA position, dental professionals often caution patients about removing amalgam fillings. The position statements of the ADA indicate that dentists are allowed to discuss the subject if the patient asks. A conventional dentist would be expected to respond to a patient's question about the safety of amalgam with information similar to that just discussed.

A Holistic View of Dental Amalgam

The holistic dentist's view of dental amalgam differs greatly from the ADA stance. Throughout the world, experts have done studies and given their opinions about the questionable safety of mercury in dental amalgams, notably for some people like the unborn or pregnant mothers (Prescrire, 2008, p. 246). The concern is about the body's ability to remove the mercury and the possibility of toxic bioburden in the cells. This bioburden can block the proper functioning of cells and can result in symptoms of serious conditions, such as autism (Geir, Kern, & Geir, 2009, p. 189).

The holistic practitioner is concerned about mercury toxicity affecting a patient in six different areas, as stated on the holistic dental website of Ronald King, a holistic dentist in Minnesota (King, 2010).

- The first concerns are neurological symptoms, such as tremors, headaches, emotional instability, anxiety, unexplained depression, and memory loss. For some patients, these symptoms resolve after amalgam removal.

- Second are cardiovascular concerns, including abnormal blood pressure and abnormal heart rhythm with improvement in symptoms after amalgam fillings are replaced.

- Third are oral disorders like bleeding gums, a metallic taste or burning sensations in the mouth, canker sores, and excessive saliva, which sometime reverse after amalgam fillings are removed.

- Fourth are immune system disorders, such as leukemia, Hodgkin's disease, multiple sclerosis, ALS, lupus erythematosis, scleroderma, and mononucleosis. In some patients, these symptoms improve after amalgam fillings are replaced.

- Fifth are gastrointestinal disorders, food sensitivities, abdominal cramps, chronic diarrhea, and constipation, all of which sometimes resolve after amalgam fillings are removed.

- Sixth are systemic disorders, such as dermatitis, thyroid disturbance, chronic fatigue, infertility, birth defects, allergies, excessive perspiration, unexplained anemia, and adrenal disease. All have been linked to dental amalgam toxicity.

Given their experiences with patients whose symptoms have lessened or disappeared after amalgam removal, holistic practitioners have linked these concerns with the presence of amalgam (Matsuzaka, Mabuchi, Nagasaka,

Yoshinari, & Inoue, 2006, p. 13). But because these are individual cases, they are considered anecdotal by the conventional dental community. These cases can be found on holistic dentists' websites. The following case is an example from the website of Ronald King.

> Female patient presents with chronic fatigue, headaches and allergies. A healthcare provider suggested she consider consulting a holistic dentist after no diagnosis could be made for her symptoms. Four months after having her amalgams removed, the headaches and chronic fatigue were gone and the usual spring allergies were improved.

Conventional dentists are not impressed with a case like this one, because the studies they rely on to verify safety show little or no risk to the participants because of the way the studies are conducted. Through a conventional lens, they fail to recognize the Eastern concepts of energy balance, meridians, and individuality.

Consider a study involving children who were tested on gross and fine motor skills over a five-year period after having amalgams placed. The study showed that no illness could be correlated with neurological, cardiovascular, gastrointestinal, oral disorders, or immunological and gastrointestinal symptoms (ADA, 2010). From the holistic perspective, for this study to be valid, the amalgam fillings must be placed on the same tooth and the same surface of the tooth for each child. Each tooth in the human mouth is on an energy line or channel that runs throughout the rest of the body affecting certain organs, nerves, and muscles. For example, the upper left six-year molar is on the same meridian as the thyroid gland (King, 2010). Fillings in different teeth affect different glands and organs. If a dental amalgam is put in this molar, the function of the thyroid may be impaired. The dysfunction of the thyroid gland may be subtle and undetectable by the instruments that are currently to measure its under-functioning. In addition, the symptoms caused in correlation with the placement of dental amalgam may not arise for fifteen, twenty, or even forty years after the fillings are put in place. And there is no way to predict when a physical or emotional trauma will alter the way the body can detoxify the affects of the mercury fumes. In other words, the harm may come years later.

The conventional interpretation of the above-mentioned study is not valid to the holistic practitioner, because fillings on different teeth cannot be compared; only ones on the same teeth are comparable. In order to compare the gross and fine motor skills of these children, therefore, a filling in the upper left first molar, for example, needs to be on all the children before the researchers can draw a conclusion. And even then, the study needs to draw conclusions about the organs that lie on that meridian, as well as the children's emotional responses, in order to be comprehensive.

To show that the amalgam had no effect on the children's motor skills, the study would also have had to show that the children perceived their experiences in the same way and their body chemistry was in the same balance. From the holistic view, it is impossible to draw valid conclusions from this study.

Rational science accepted as valid by the ADA describes measurements and draws conclusions, but does not evaluate all the necessary parameters identified by the holistic approach. It does not take into account that each human subject is unique and one cannot evaluate them as being the same. Therefore, holistic practitioners do not generalize. Human bodies are not machines that can reproduce results in the same manner each time. The human body reacts differently to influences in the environment on a physiological, mental, and emotional level. Individuals simply cannot be seen as the same.

Material Choices

Patients rely on their dentists to decide what kind of materials to use in making a crown, bridge, or denture/partial denture. The dentist judges whether the location of the tooth requires a more durable material; he also determines the aesthetic look of the material, how practical the material is to use, and the cost, and then makes a recommendation.

The holistic dentist takes into consideration other criteria, like the potential harmfulness to the patient, when making the decision about what material to use based on the following concepts (King, 2010):

- First, the holistic dentist considers a patient's individual response when constructing a crown, bridge, or partial. Patients are individuals and they may react to a material to which no other patient has shown an allergic response. A holistic dentist makes sure to update each patient's full medical history before using dental materials in order to identify any new allergies. The holistic practitioner knows that chronic symptoms can signal an underlying material or food allergy that brings an adverse reaction. The holistic dentist then discusses the choice of materials with the patient.

- Second, the holistic dentist considers allergies. Some patients with multiple allergies may choose to have blood tests to identify sensitivity to dental materials.

Labs specializing in dental sensitivity tests compare all the materials used in a dental office to the individual's blood to detect any allergies to the different substances. The lab then sends a report to the dentist showing the least reactive materials that are compatible with the individual.

- The third consideration is toxicity: Some dental materials may be toxic for certain patients who already have a compromised immune system or a chronic illness. Qualified professionals can determine nontoxic alternatives through blood test so as not to worsen the patient's health and increase the toxic bioburden on the patient's system.

- Fourth, the holistic dentist will consider if there are interference fields. Holistic practitioners recognize that some materials can disrupt the flow of energy in the meridians. Chronic interference can result in ill health or a worsening condition. This may limit the number of material choices available.

- Fifth is electro galvanism. When metals combine in the mouth with saliva, an electrical current is emitted that may cause pain, dry mouth, a metallic taste, redness, fluid accumulation, and dysfunction of the organs on the meridian that runs through the tooth on which the material was placed. The following scenario illustrates material sensitivity by oral galvanism.

Female patient presented for treatment with complaints of constant coughing since a partial denture was placed.

The partial was constructed of metal and acrylic materials. The patient had consulted two conventional dentists. She wondered if there was a connection between the coughing and the placement of the new partial (King, 2010).

The two conventional dentists both discounted any connection to galvanism. Instead, they concluded that the symptoms were due to the fact that the space for the tongue was inadequate and the size of the teeth on the partial prevented adequate movement, triggering the coughing. The patient then consulted a dentist with a holistic approach for another opinion.

The holistic dentist, however, suspected oral galvanism. The patient was instructed to go without the partial and watch for any symptoms. There were none. To confirm that her symptoms were due to galvanism and not something else, the dentist instructed the patient to put a coin in her mouth. After trying the coin, the coughing returned. Based on this simple experiment, the dentist made a new nonmetal partial. The constant coughing subsided after the patient used the new nonmetal partial (King, 2010).

Seeing the Individual

The main point dividing the conventional approach and the holistic approach is the concept of individuality. The conventional dental practitioner and the governing body, the ADA, rely on science that draws conclusions from studies of groups of people on which to base their protocols for dental practice. The holistic dentist knows, based on Eastern concepts, that one simply cannot draw conclusions about the effect of dental materials on an individual based on studies that draw conclusions about groups of individuals. Everyone reacts differently because bodies have different biochemical makeups, which are affected by a person's mental, emotional, and physical environment.

Using a group of individuals to see if they have any adverse reactions to dental amalgam is like trying to compare the interior condition of two homes in a city. Each home over a period of time is exposed to the same external weather conditions and temperature. What happens inside the home, however, is what needs to be taken into account. If one is kept at seventy degrees year round and humidity is kept low, the condition of that home will be different than the home in which the temperature is kept at 85 degrees with no humidity control. In Minnesota during the winter, the second home will be dry; in the summer, it will be damp. Over a period of five years, there may be few differences, but over twenty years, there will be a difference in the interior condition of the two homes.

Other factors come into consideration also. How are the two homes maintained? One may be kept clean while the other is allowed to collect dust, dirt, mold, and mildew. One home may have pets that contribute to air quality and the other home has air purifiers. I could go on and on with additional qualifiers, but the point is clear: They cannot be compared in a study. While the two homes can be compared as to changes to come to valid conclusions shows ignorance of the many variables overlooked. The homes and how they are cared for is very complex. People are also complex.

The same is true in studies that the ADA relies on to validate safety claims. There are too many variables to consider and accurately compare when studying a person's reaction to dental materials. Valid conclusions cannot be made without considering all the components that make up the individual. And the patient may not react in a month or year. It may be a dozen or more years when they react because of events that happen preventing their body from detoxing properly.

We can see once again that the conventional dentist and the holistic dentist differ in their views of how dentistry affects the human body. One relies on scientific studies conducted by examiners using the Cartesian-Newtonian method of evaluation; the other uses information from scientific studies as well as anecdotal cases to draw conclusions. In this country, we have been educated to accept scientific proof as trustworthy. Scientific studies using a method based on Eastern philosophy are difficult to conduct because the individual patients' reactions are all different.

Comparing the two approaches by using the same measurement tool is also impossible. Conventional dentistry measures things that are objective and can be seen. Holistic dentistry uses subjective tools to measure improvement. For example, the holistic dentist may use the patient's perceptions or improvement of symptoms in the whole body as a valid measurement that there is improvement after mercury fillings are removed. The conventional dentists might use blood tests or urine tests as measurements. The holistic dentists might use these objective tools also, but the patient's perceptions of improvement are equally as important.

Another example: Just as you cannot measure electrical current in the same way you measure liquids, you cannot measure energy medicine just with the objective assessment tools that conventional medicine advocates. You are trying to measure the seen and the unseen with the same tools. There simply is no way to compare the measurement of cups of liquid and watts of electricity. They are different and conclusions must be made about each separately. Holistic dentistry and conventional dentistry cannot be measured in the same way. One treats symptoms (conventional) while the other looks for a cause (holistic). From the holistic vantage point, it makes sense to use the good of both and deliver the best care to patients who trust their dentists.

FOUR

FACTORS PREVENTING
THE INTEGRATION OF
PHILOSOPHIES

A coherence criterion of truth means all facts are in proper
relationship to one another being pertinent, systematic,
integrated and consistent. If new facts arise they must be
understood and integrated as relevant into the whole. The
problem may be, however, that man's limitations may
prevent him from obtaining all the facts of an experience.
The question is can there be equally coherent systems each
containing all the facts of an experience?

SAHAKIAN, 2005, P. 11

The case for integrating the Eastern concepts of individuality, balance, and meridian theory into dentistry is
compelling. Patients are seen first as individuals who may
not respond to conventional dental treatment and materials all in the same way. The dental practitioner will look at

the patient's mouth as a reflection of the rest of the body, with all the parts interconnected. A holistic dentist will see something like gum disease as indicating an imbalance in the body. In a case like this, he may counsel his patients on nutrition or refer the patient to conventional dental specialists or natural practitioners, such as naturopaths, homeopaths, acupuncturists, chiropractors, and so forth.

From the holistic point of view, unexplained illness like chronic headaches, pain in the jaw, or even other body illness are seen as symptoms of underlying causes to be solved by cranial sacral, cranial adjustments, acupuncture, Rolfing, and other holistic techniques. The dentist and auxiliaries help patients eliminate chronic health complaints that may be related to the individual's dentistry or remain unsolved by medical doctors. Dental patients can be referred to other practitioners to find the cause of disease, rather than just have their symptoms treated. Patients will benefit from the coordination of dentists, medical doctors, and alternative practitioners to get to the source of their diseases.

The question remains why the dental profession, organized for 150 years, has not integrated Eastern concepts into dentistry when it appears patients can benefit from doing so. Are holistic and conventional dentistry both coherent systems, and can they together serve the population for the good of all? To find an answer, I will discuss the assumptions the ADA and the holistic-minded dentists make in delivering care to the American public.

First, one must ask the following questions: What criterion for validity are they using to substantiate their claims? Can they work in harmony to better serve the population? If so, what are the factors that prevent integration?

The ADA's number one assumption is that the dental practices and protocols it has established are generally safe for dental patients. Holistic dentists claim, however, that some of the ADA's dental practices and protocols are unsafe. Second, the ADA relies on scientific studies in peer-reviewed publications to prove safety, and any improvement of a patient's symptoms from a holistic treatment is seen as due to the placebo effect. The holistic dentist relies on individual case histories to show there is evidence of harm. By looking at each approach to dentistry, conventional and holistic, separately, I will discuss the way they verify their claims and whether or not their claims are valid.

Assumptions of the ADA

Anyone can go to the ADA website and get information about dental procedures and materials. There are two easily recognizable options on the ADA website, one for professionals and one for the public. Both have information about dental amalgams. This excerpt is from the public page on dental amalgams.

> Used by dentists for more than a century, dental amalgam is the most thoroughly researched and tested restorative material among all those in use . . . mercury in amalgam combines with other metals to render it stable and safe for use in filling teeth. Questions have arisen about the safety of dental amalgam relating to its mercury content. The major U.S. and international scientific and health bodies, including the National Institutes of Health, the U.S. Public Health Service, the Centers for Disease Control and Prevention, the Food and Drug Administration and the World Health Organization have been satisfied that dental

amalgam is a safe, reliable and effective restorative material.

Amalgam fillings, like other filling materials, are considered biocompatible—they are
well tolerated by patients with only rare occurrences of allergic response (p. 3094).

Upon reading this description of dental amalgam as
a filling option, one may assume that the safety of dental
amalgam has been thoroughly investigated. However, if
one looks under the options for the dental professional,
one will find contradictory information. The ADA
council on scientific affairs recommends precautions for
dental professionals: "The ADA has long recognized the
importance of observing proper mercury hygiene practices
for the safety of dental professionals" (ADA, 2010).
Under the title "Practice Implications," it states, "These
recommendations are intended to provide guidance to the
dental practitioner in ensuring the safety of personnel who
handle dental amalgam and in minimizing the release of
mercury into the dental office environment" (p. 1498).
In addition to the above statement by the ADA, the following is recommended for the handling and disposing of
amalgam in the precautions for waste management:

The "Best Management Practices (BMPs)
for Amalgam Waste" are a series of amalgam
waste handling and disposal practices that
include but are not limited to initiating bulk
mercury collection programs, using chair side
traps and vacuum collection, inspecting and
cleaning traps, and recycling or using a commer-
cial waste disposal service to dispose of the
amalgam collected (ADA, 2010).

After reading the above, a reader may become confused. Two major questions arise. First, are they really safe for everyone? What if I am one of the *rare* persons with a reaction? Second, if dental amalgams are so safe, why is a waste-management practice needed to protect the provider and the environment?

Safe for Everyone?

The ADA claims that combining mercury with other alloys renders it stable and safe to use in the mouth. It also states that the Food and Drug Administration (FDA) is satisfied that it is safe. The FDA claimed in a literature review, "Mercury exposure from dental amalgam is not believed by USPHS agencies and WHO (World Health Organization) to represent levels associated with adverse health effects in humans, including sensitive populations" (ADA, 2010). If this is true, then why have concern for dental professionals? One may argue that exposure to radiation for a dental x-ray would be bad for the dentist if he or she held the x-ray for every patient, because of the accumulative effects of the radiation in the body tissues. It also makes logical sense that if a dentist's skin is in contact with the newly placed amalgam of every patient he treats, he may then be at risk.

If amalgam is a stable alloy once hardened, then why the concern about handling hardened amalgam from plumbing traps that need cleaning? And if amalgam is safe, what difference does it make if it is flushed into the environment? After all, as stated earlier, "mercury in amalgam combines with other metals to render it stable and safe." The ADA states that "because dentists are good stewards of the environment, it is prudent to limit the release of any dental amalgam waste to the environment" (ADA,

2010). Why doesn't this also mean the environment of the human body?

I understand the implications of the ADA's position to be these: If amalgam is safe to put in a patient's mouth, it is also safe to flush into the sewer. Or, if these fillings are affecting the environment, then dental amalgam is constantly affecting the environment in the human body.

Of course it might be argued that the environment of planet earth cannot eliminate the toxic effect of mercury as the body can. In the FDA literature I've seen, dental amalgams were reported to be safe, including for "sensitive populations" (ADA, 2010). The ADA site for the public states, "Amalgam fillings, like other filling materials, are considered biocompatible—they are well tolerated by patients with only rare occurrences of allergic response" (ADA, 2010). So what does this position mean for the American public who are sensitive to dental amalgam? There seems to be little concern by the ADA for the sensitive person who is unable to eliminate this waste.

The argument by the ADA contains additional flaws. There is a general consensus that amalgam is safe to use because it has been used for more than 150 years. It is the custom of dentists who look to the ADA for guidance to use amalgam. If this is their criteria for truth, then Chinese medicine should be used, because it has been around for three thousand years. Second, the pragmatist would say about dental amalgam, "It works!" But does it really? It does fill a cavity and is easy to use, especially on children. But is there more to be considered here? Given that there are dental professionals who are educated in the same schools as the dental professionals in the ADA who dispute the safety of amalgam, one might be inclined to ask if dental amalgam really works for every individual.

Last, the ADA argument is not coherent. It does not consider all relevant factors. In particular, it does not consider all the facts. Case histories of patients harmed by dental amalgam demonstrate this. Many holistic colleagues have observed harm to patients from their dental amalgams and publish their findings. For example, over thirty years ago, Hal Huggins wrote a controversial book called *It's All in Your Head: The Link between Mercury Amalgams and Illness*. Huggins is seen as a warrior by holistic dental professionals and as the devil himself by the ADA. He, however, is not the first warrior professing the dangers of mercury use in dental fillings over the last 150 years. There have been others who have championed the idea that mercury in the form of dental amalgam causes slight to severe consequences for some members of the American public. Why hasn't something been done to acknowledge all studies here and abroad out of concern for the sensitive dental population?

Anecdotal Evidence

Hal Huggins relates the stories of two cases involving dental amalgam. Their uniqueness shows how difficult it is to acquire this information from a scientific study and the importance of treating each individual patient as a study all in themselves. The patients and their families endured immense suffering due to something as simple as their dental work interfering with their health.

Jan was a seventeen-year-old who had experienced severe chest pains when having her teeth filled with amalgam. Her dentist told her she was just anxious about being at the dental office. She then suffered attacks of chest pains and severe acne over the next few months. She went from medical doctor to medical doctor only to be told it was all in her head and she needed to be institutionalized in a mental hospital. By the time she found Dr. Huggins, she had been to the emergency room a dozen times and was unable to be the good student she once had been. Dr. Huggins found her blood tests were not conclusive, but at the urging of Jan's parents, removed her dental amalgams. Four days later, she was able to return to school, complete two semesters of work, and graduate without the previous symptoms that had limited her life (Huggins, 1993, p. 12).

In the second case, eleven-year-old Susan was experiencing seizures every fifteen minutes. She was given only three months to live when her parents brought her to Dr. Huggins to remove the amalgam fillings from her teeth. The process was logistically tricky to complete: He had to administer the anesthesia, remove the amalgams, and replace them with composite tooth-colored fillings between the seizures. It took two dental assistants, the child's father, and Dr. Huggins to complete the procedures and to prevent her from falling out of the chair and hurting herself during the treatment. Six days later, she woke up on December 25, the seizures gone, and she was able to navigate the stairs of her home by herself to experience Christmas Day. She had no more seizures and in the spring was videotaped participating in track events (p. 15). The comment by the ADA on hearing the report of this case was, "We are not impressed" (p. 16).

Science Showing Harm

For the first half of my dental hygiene career, I trusted my training and relied on the science my profession accepted as valid. Ever since my introduction to energy medicine, however, I now question and am suspicious of the concepts I was taught to rely upon as the truth. In his book *Understanding Behaviorism: Behavior, Culture, and Evolution,* William Baum says, "Science is not about the truth, however, but rather about a systematic way to pass information from generation to generation" (2005, p. 27). As a healthcare provider, I thought science was about proven and verified facts. To me, this means that all is taken into account when deciding what is valid. Some will question my interpretation of Baum's words; however, as a homeopath and a holistic dental hygienist, this quote has the ring of truth in it. I now interpret science as a way we discover information and pass it on to others. The information gained is a picture of a moment in time under certain controls, but not necessarily the whole truth.

Over the years, I have witnessed dental patients who have been harmed by the materials and procedures we use in dentistry, in spite of the fact they are backed by science. While the profession is supposed to "do no harm," we clearly are. The ADA code of ethics states in section two principles regarding nonmalfeasance ("do no harm"):

> This principle expresses the concept that professionals have a duty to protect the patient from harm. Under this principle, the dentist's primary obligations include keeping knowledge and skills current, knowing one's own limitations and when to refer to a specialist or other professional, and knowing when and under what circumstances delegation of patient care to auxiliaries is appropriate (ADA, 2010).

The ADA and conventional medicine in general often see cases like those presented by Huggins, if they recognize them at all, as involving the placebo effect, with a placebo being a therapeutic effect as a result of the patient believing the treatment is effective. While the ADA is not impressed by these cases because they are anecdotal accounts, neither is it impressed by the scientific studies conducted by Boyd Haley, a professor of chemistry at the University of Kentucky and chairman of the chemistry department since 1996. The ADA has refuted his claims, as well as Hal Huggins. His research centers on biochemical and biomedical problems involving control at the molecular level and in biological systems regulated by protein-nucleotide interactions. His studies include the effect of mercury on tissues and some biochemical changes found in nerve cells in Alzheimer's disease and autism (Haley, 2001).

Haley concludes that mercury from dental amalgams can have a cumulative toxic effect on the body and possibly be a potential cause of autism and Alzheimer's disease (2001). He poses some serious concerns and his studies, viewed by the American consumer, might trigger the following questions: If there is a remote possibility this is true, doesn't it make sense to review the reasons dentists still use dental amalgam, and to stop using it until there is more conclusive evidence of its safety for use in all patients' mouths? Or at least shouldn't the ADA warn the public about the possibility that some people may be sensitive to dental amalgams? As I stated earlier, the ADA argument is not coherent and ignores facts of scientific evidence by Boyd Haley and anecdotal evidence by Hal Huggins. The organization has not integrated the helpful information discussed here into their advised protocols and principles to deliver more comprehensive holistic care.

Unlike some of their colleagues, holistic dental professionals assume that dentistry is not always safe, based on individual case histories, scientific evidence, and other countries' positions on safety of dental amalgam.

In fact, research on this topic is available from other countries. Canada, Norway, Sweden, Britain, Germany, and Denmark all advise dentists against using amalgam fillings on pregnant women (Larsen, 2008). And one Canadian study by K. Aminzadeh entitled "Dental amalgam and multiple sclerosis: a systemic review and meta-analysis" concludes that additional studies are needed to definitely rule out a link between amalgam and multiple sclerosis. Such studies from foreign sources suggest there may be a connection between certain illness and the use of dental amalgams, and that further study is needed (Aminzadeh & Etminan, 2007).

Peer Review

John Dodes, in "The amalgam controversy: An evidence-based analysis," reviewed studies in peer-reviewed and non-peer-reviewed publications. He contends that there are methodological errors in the anti-amalgam literature and concludes the evidence is compelling that dental amalgam is safe and effective. He states, "Dentists *should* educate patients and other healthcare professionals who may be *mistakenly concerned* about amalgam safety" (Dodes, 2001, p. 348). Conventional dentists like John Dodes come to the conclusion that amalgams are safe. Studies that support this claim are relied on because they have used the scientific method and they are published in peer-reviewed journals. This is the gold standard for truth and validity in conventional dentistry. These studies don't consider all the pertinent facts from all sources, however, and conclusions using words like "should" and "mistakenly concerned" show bias and judgment on the researcher's part. He demonstrates attachment to the ADA claim of dental amalgam safety by the words he used. He could have stated, from his review, dentists can use amalgam without concern of ill harm to patients.

What Do Other Scientists Say about Holistic Therapies?

R. Barker Bausell, former research director at National Institutes of Health–funded Complementary and Alternative Medicine Specialized Research Center, looked at the research of holistic therapies in his book *Snake Oil Science*. His goal was to investigate whether holistic therapies work. Bausell reviewed research methods and found that holistic therapies work temporarily and weakly. He said that holistic studies are poorly designed and some of the results are placebo effect. In contrast, he discusses research from respected journals that employed placebo controls. The results show that holistic therapies do not have positive results any more than random chance (Bausell, 2007).

The Placebo Effect

Holistic practitioners acknowledge the placebo effect may be responsible for improvement while treating clients. However, most homeopaths who practice classical homeopathy, the method used by the founder Samuel Hahneman, relate accounts of treating children and pets to counter concerns that all positive results from homeopathic treatments result from the placebo effect. These "clients" know nothing of the placebo effect, and at the time of receiving the remedy, probably think the caregiver is actually being mean. And even if not, a small child in discomfort receiving a homeopathic remedy will probably not think, "This will make me better."

The scientific method is not able to assess the complexity of the individual nature of all persons in the study, nor can it predict if a response is placebo effect. One can draw some conclusions from the information in a scientific

double-blind placebo controlled study; however, the holistic practitioner knows the method used cannot accurately
assess why energy therapies like homeopathy or acupuncture work.

Scientific Research and Holistic Therapies

Researchers have done scientific studies on holistic
therapies, but these studies have produced varied results,
largely because of the individual natures of the people studied. For example, if ten people with eczema go to the same
homeopath, they will in all likelihood receive ten different
remedies. A practitioner would prescribe remedies based on
the totality of a person's symptoms, how he thinks, how he
feels, how he relate to others, and his physical conditions;
it is unlikely that any two people would be the same on
all of these scores. If ten patients went to a medical doctor complaining of eczema, on the other hand, they would
probably receive the same prescription, a cortisone cream
to control or eliminate the symptoms. So when it comes
to quantifying the results of homeopathic treatments, the
many variables make it difficult to come to the kinds of
conclusions accepted by the medical and research community. Some practitioners in holistic disciplines, however,
feel compelled to try and prove the effectiveness of holistic
treatments by applying the scientific method to gain acceptance. This causes them to generalize rather than apply the
treatment on the individual.

One such homeopathic scientific study was conducted
on infants in Nicaragua who suffered from diarrhea
(Jacobs, Jonas, Jimenez-Perez, & Crothers, 2003). Four
homeopathic remedies that commonly work for diarrhea
were used to treat infants with the condition. From the
symptoms presented by each infant, the practitioner prescribed the best of the four remedies. While this study is
scientifically based, many classical homeopaths (trained to

practice using one remedy at a time) would be opposed to using homeopathy in this manner, because it is a watered-down approach of the art. In this study, the practitioner was really treating symptoms rather than the person. In other words he was treating the disease the infant had rather than treating the person who had the disease. According to classical homeopathy, the practitioner should have been finding the cause of the diarrhea, since the diarrhea was a symptom of the underlying cause problem. The classical homeopath would rather evaluate each individual child on the mental, emotional, and physical levels and then prescribe a remedy matching their symptoms. In all probability, each child would receive a different remedy to treat the diarrhea (Vithoulkas, 1980).

Energy-based medicine looks for the cause of the discomfort. Conventional treatment in many cases only treats the symptoms. What is needed is a coherent view to treat both to make the patient well. In the context of dental treatments, for example, if the dental patient has cavities frequently, we need to find the cause. Treating the patient with fluoride, education on preventing cavities, and a filling is half of the prescription. The patient needs counseling on nutrition, but the practitioner should also look into the person's body chemistry, susceptibility to dental decay, and the metabolism. While scientific studies may offer some general conclusions, they do not take into consideration the many variables that anecdotal evidence can more accurately address. Using information from both is necessary to arrive at valid conclusions.

Integration Procrastination

Why hasn't the integration of Eastern and Western medical wisdom happened? Could it be that economics or the traditions of the ADA as a patriarchal institution have prevented integration? Or do dental schools tend to choose students who have been shaped behaviorally and will conform to practice dentistry in a certain manner? Are there psychological factors of the intellect and ego at play, or is it a matter of the spirit of the conventional dental professional disrupted by greed, jealousy, and closed mindedness (the three poisons), as the Tibetans believe?

In researching this topic, I came across a true story of how human nature plays a role in this dilemma. Aversion to accepting a new idea or person has been around for many years. In Will Frackelton's book *The Sagebrush Dentist,* I was struck by the politics of turf protection back in the late 1800s. Frackelton's book is a biography of his early years as a dentist going to a small town in the wild West upon graduation. The local sheriff was not pleased when Frackelton came to town, because his friend was a dentist. Frackelton's presence meant that his friend would have a competitor, and it took some time before the newcomer was accepted (Frackleton & Seely, 1947). It is human nature to approach something or someone new with caution, and the same is probably true of holistic dentistry. Also, integrating holistic concepts might suggest to the public that conventional dentistry has done something wrong.

But this may be true. Many books are written on the subject of mercury poisoning and how the mercury in dental fillings leaches out into the mouths of patients with the potential to cause harm to general health. Study after study is offered as proof of harm, as well as anecdotal evidence of harm to individuals.

There are a few studies that the ADA refers to on their

website under the topics for professionals that refer the safety of using dental amalgam. None of the studies provided by the ADA for its professionals to review take into consideration the patient as an individual with an immune system that is unique. All the studies are of a one-size-fits-all approach.

As a dental hygienist, classical homeopath, health coach, and former educator, I feel compelled to question what prevents my colleagues from seeing the possible consequences of this powerful neurotoxin on the human brain. While one person's body may detoxify the mercury after an amalgam restoration, another person with a chronic health condition or a compromised mental emotional state might not detoxify the mercury as well. Patients are individuals and need to be treated as such. Each person has a unique body with its own set of variables. In the last century and a half, the American public has put trust in the ADA body to protect their health. I believe part of the resistance to integration of holistic concepts may be the history of the ADA itself.

Is the Answer about History?

Let's begin with a look at how the ADA got its roots. In the mid-1800s, the ADA was preceded by an organization called the American Society of Dental Surgeons. This group was concerned about the effects of mercury in the silver fillings being used at the time and resolved to eliminate them from the practice of dentistry. There was evidence at that time regarding neurological effects of mercury poisoning in the fillings (Wynbrandt, 1998).

In the late 1850s, however, a new society was formed, the ADA, the one we know today. It was formed to allow dentists to use mercury fillings for their patients, as well as set standards for practice and education (Wynbrandt, 1998). Mercury fillings were cheaper than other alternatives, such as gold, and easy to use because the prepared tooth did not need to be kept dry. These reasons are still referred to today, even though there is a mountain of evidence suggesting dental amalgam might be harmful to patients.

What about Politics and Economics?

There were political factors, too. The ADA was assigned two patents on the composition of dental amalgam and the amalgamation process. The ADA claims they never received any compensation from the patents. Private companies make dental amalgam. The ADA denies that it controls these companies. Today, even though the patents are expired, one can only suspect the possible politics of not wanting to admit they held patents on this potentially harmful material as discussed earlier. In spite of the denial that it has power over amalgam manufacturers, the ADA certainly wields power by regulating the manufacturing industry and by requiring dentists to carry out the dental placement of amalgam.

In the 1990s several dentists were investigated and lost their licenses for supporting amalgam removal because of its toxicity in some patients. The ADA stated positions on the materials and their use in an accepted dental practice. The position of the ADA today is that amalgam fillings—fifty percent of which are mercury—are biologically inactive.

Those who advocate for the removal of mercury from amalgam or the discontinued use of "silver fillings" like Hal Huggins of Colorado, profess and establish a good

argument for the harm that occurs in the mouths of millions of Americans. But one can only imagine what the cost
would be to the ADA and its member dentists, not to men-
tion the fall from grace the association might experience in
the eyes of the American public, if the ADA were to admit
amalgam's harmful effects. The ADA and member dentists
risk losing influence and power by admitting harm.

If dental amalgam was conclusively determined by the
FDA to be potentially hazardous, the backlash from the
American public would make the lawsuits over tobacco
and asbestos look very small in comparison. A smaller pro-
portion of the public smokes or is exposed to asbestos than
has amalgam fillings. Indeed, most Americans have dental
fillings and millions have dental amalgam fillings. To protect its standing, the ADA must defend the use of amalgam
as safe. To admit otherwise might bankrupt the institution
and member dentists from the demand by the public for
reparations.

The Struggle for Acceptance

New ideas and theories, as well as the people who
profess them, struggle for acceptance into the conventional
dental establishment. George Collis, inventor of the Collis
Curve toothbrush, is a prime example. His revolutionary
idea of a brush that would remove plaque from all sides
of the teeth at once was met with opposition by the dental
community and the ADA. It didn't help that he was not a
member of the ADA at the time.

Collis thought that getting the ADA's seal of approval,
a measurement of safety and efficiency, would give cred-
ibility to his invention. When he contacted the ADA in the
mid-1980s to apply for the seal, he was told that there was

no seal for toothbrushes. However, a few months later, a representative from the ADA was on the Phil Donahue talk show discussing a new toothbrush called the "Reach" toothbrush, and commented that it had the seal from the ADA (Collis, 2007).

Once the ADA admitted there was a seal for toothbrushes, Collis applied for it. By this time, the Collis Curve toothbrush had been on the market for over five years. He had dozens of letters of support for the brush from faithful users. Also, some clinical results were documented in his practice and scientific studies were commencing. Surely, he thought, this would be enough to attain the seal.

In October of 1984 a study was published in the *Journal of Dentistry for Children* called "Give your teeth a hug: A simplified brushing technique for children" (Avery, 1984). This study showed positive results for the curved bristle brush. It easily gave children an advantage over the straight bristle by brushing all surfaces of the teeth at once. There was little possibility of missing areas, a common occurrence when children tried to master the straight-bristle toothbrush.

In November 1987, a study was published about the effectiveness of the straight-bristle toothbrush compared to the curved-bristle brush (Shory, Mitchell, & Jamison, 1987). The results showed that the Collis Curve was as effective as the straight bristle. Collis submitted the Shory study to the ADA. The ADA rejected his application, including other evidence, saying that the supporting study was anecdotal and did not meet the protocol. Collis's request to get the protocol was met with a denial to release it. How, then, could Collis ever make sure that his supporting studies met the ADA's protocol if he was not allowed to see it?

In 1988, another study was published in the *Journal of Dentistry for Children* entitled "The curved-bristle toothbrush: an aid for the handicapped population" (Williams,

Johnson, & Schuman, 1988). Once again, the ADA rejected this study, as it had the rest. It said the study did not meet the protocol. When asked for the protocol, the ADA refused. Collis's frustration was growing, and his attempt to get his brush accepted by his profession seemed futile. He then decided to sue the ADA.

Suing the ADA meant getting an attorney from Illinois and depositions of the ADA staff attorneys. Collis, his wife, and his daughter, Jane Collis Gonzales, went to the deposition. The judge who reviewed the case to determine if it would go to trial stated that Dr. Collis had been given the runaround by the ADA. He ordered the ADA to conduct another study at its own cost. The study was to be completed within thirty days. The results would determine if Collis's invention would receive the seal of acceptance. The judge also gave the ADA the option to release their confidential files to Collis's representative to prepare for a trial, instead of doing a study. The ADA chose to do the study (Collis, 2007).

Following the celebration in Collis's office over this great victory, the staff was surprised when a phone call came from Richard Meckstroff. He had conducted research on the brush in the 1980s and the ADA had just called him to conduct the new study. Even more surprising was the response he got when he requested the ADA's protocol. The ADA told him that there was no protocol for studies submitted for the seal of acceptance. For years, the ADA's big bureaucracy had played with Dr. Collis, a small inventor with a revolutionary idea. But just as David slew Goliath, Collis won over the big giant. The new study, of course, revealed positive results for the curved-bristle toothbrush. However, the ADA had one more obstacle for George Collis.

Meckstroff called Dr. Collis after the study was complete and shared with him that one person in the study had an adverse reaction—some minor bleeding—to the brush.

Shortly after that, Dr. Collis received a letter from the ADA attorney asking him to sign a form saying that Collis would not receive the seal if even one person had an adverse reaction. This time, Dr. Collis was ahead of the ADA, and of course refused to sign the form. Finally, the Collis Curve received the seal of acceptance, a great victory after the Collis family's great struggle.

This story is an example of how the ADA controls what happens regarding the acceptance of practices and products in dentistry. It also makes me question the science the ADA is willing to accept. The Collis brush was researched by several independent researchers with no interest in the product other than to study its effectiveness. The ADA rejected the protocols used in the Collis Curve studies and then later admitted they had no standard or protocol of their own by which to evaluate brushes. The public relies on the institution of the ADA to help protect them, but in the process, as this story demonstrates, some of the best ideas may have to struggle to benefit patients.

Psychology

While the ADA's history may supply the answer that prevents the integration of holistic concepts into dentistry, could resistance also be the mindset of individual dentists? Student dentists are admitted based on their intellectual abilities to go through the rigors of the dental education. Ambika Wauters, in her book *Chakras and Their Archetypes: Uniting Energy Awareness and Spiritual Growth,* discusses Carl Jung's intellectual archetype. The intellectual spends a lot of time analyzing, or using left-brain thinking. This is a great activity for dental professionals to exercise in order to become critical thinkers when delivering care;

however, according to Wauters, intellectuals "constantly rely on habitual or mechanical responses to new situations that limit possibilities for expansion" (Wauters, 1997, p. 129). Why is this the case? It is much safer to rely on the familiar than the unknown, and dentists are taught to base their decisions on information from secondary sources, like their professional association, rather than make their own observations and trust their own intuitions when treating patients. To be fair, this is partly understandable, considering their dental licenses could be at stake if they stray too far from the protocols of the governing body. That dental professionals spend their careers rationalizing their behavior is what the ADA or state boards expect of them.

From My Viewpoint

I see the prevention of integration of holistic concepts into dentistry to be a result of the historical customs of the ADA and the shaping of individual dentists to do as they must in order to keep their licenses and make their livings. It is easier to go along with the system rather than oppose it with other observations and beliefs. For if they explore possibilities contrary to ADA expectations and what they learn makes sense, they would be compelled to make decisions to take action and integrate these changes into their practices. But it is easier to stay in a familiar place than move into the unfamiliar.

The ADA has for 150 years denied that amalgams are harmful. The reason, I believe, is multifaceted. One facet is economic. As I stated earlier, to admit that amalgams have harmed patients might lead to the financial ruin of the member dentists and to their authority. Patients might feel victimized by the power of the institution and may demand reparations. Dentists may be accused of being greedy and closed-minded. A second is ethical. Dentists would have to admit they violated their ethical code to do no harm. It is easier to stay in the safety zone of conventional practice than to risk disturbing one's conscience. Still another facet is psychological: To admit harm would mean that dentists would need to change their entire belief system, revising and reestablishing relationships with colleagues, staff, and patients.

In addition to the dental amalgam controversy, other controversial topics, such as root canal therapy, cavitations, oral galvanism, bridges, and fluoride, might compound the outcry by the public. I believe many dental professionals are aware of the possibility of harm to the patient, but don't know how to get out of the predicament. It is easier to see the cases of harmed patients as only a few than to admit it may be a bigger problem.

Adding to the dilemma is the history of anti-amalgam dentists under scrutiny by the ADA and individual state boards since 1990. *Sixty Minutes* reporter Morley Safer interviewed a number of patients whose health improved when their mercury fillings were removed. He also reported the case of a New York dentist, Joel Berger, who lost his license for his anti-mercury views (Sullivan, 2004). Hal Huggins, whose work I cited earlier, lost his license to practice dentistry in 1996 in Colorado. Gary Jacobsen, a Minnesota dentist, gave up his license after repeated costly investigations into his manner of practicing. It became clear to licensed dentists throughout the country that they must be careful discussing their positions on mercury (Sullivan, 2004).

While there is no gag order on discussing the amalgam filling controversy, the position statement from the ADA is that dentists can discuss it if the patient asks about amalgam harm and removal of fillings (ADA, 2010). When the patient asks about the dangers of amalgam fillings, more than likely the response from the dentist will be a confirmation of the ADA position on dental amalgam. After all, the dentist is under the jurisdiction of the state board, which in turn abides by the ADA philosophy.

From my view, the code of ethics to do no harm means to do no harm to any individual. If there is even the slightest possibility that amalgam may harm even a few people, the situation warrants investigation and the further prevention of harm for all dental patients. Ignorance of any viable alternative philosophy and mere options are no excuses for shirking the responsibility the dental professional has to the American public. The dental profession is, however, made up of intellectuals who rely on responding in the same manner as they have for 150 years. Their peers confirm that their philosophy is valid. They resort to justifying their position by quoting the science they have judged correct, and discount the other studies that conclude that amalgam causes harm as anecdotal or somehow faulty.

PART
II

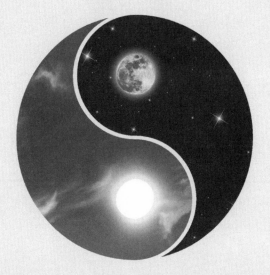

MAKING DENTISTRY WHOLE

FIVE

THE LOOK OF
INTEGRATED DENTISTRY

Along the way we face moral dilemmas. Even Charles Lindberg chose beauty over power and commerce when he said, 'If I have to choose, I would rather have birds than airplanes.' Perhaps we can have both.

FRED AMRAM (2008)

Holistic dentists rely on the philosophy of holism. They know the whole is greater than the sum of the parts. Because they, like their conventional colleagues, are trained in a reductive method, they acknowledge the importance of the parts, but they also believe that one cannot predict the behavior of a system, no matter how much data is available. In observing individual case histories, they see patients reacting to materials, like amalgam, and procedures in an adverse way. They can only assume that the patient's dentistry is the cause if, for example, amalgams are removed and the patient's symptoms disappear.

Conventional dentists operate from naïve realism: "If

I see it, I believe it." They can't put any faith in things that they are unable to describe or quantify. While they often cannot explain certain variables, surrendering to principles of energy medicine is not within their scope of reality. In contrast, the holistic dentist believes there are truths beyond the scope of the senses. This is the key to understanding the differences in the two groups.

It is easy for me to understand and accept holistic dentistry because of my background in energy medicine and homeopathy, and because I am the daughter of a dowser. I grew up knowing some things cannot be explained by science, but that doesn't mean they don't or can't work. The arguments that holistic dentists make are coherent from my viewpoint, as they look at all the parts from their conventional training and integrate knowledge they have acquired regarding holism in alternative and complimentary therapies.

Strengths of Conventional and Holistic Dentistry

Conventional dentists rely on reducing things to individual parts, while the holistic dentist sees all the parts and how they interrelate and contribute to the whole. This is precisely where I think the two can exist and complement one another. I concede that many services that conventional dentistry provides are beneficial. Holistic dentistry also offers valuable services. They each do some things well. To acknowledge one perspective's strengths from the point of view of the other could provide the best service for the public. For this to happen, however, the conventional dentist must recognize and acknowledge that a percentage of the population is possibly harmed by their dentistry, and there is a need to incorporate other ideas when delivering the best care to dental patients.

A Summary of the Two World Views.

Strengths of Conventional Dentistry	Strengths of Holistic Dentistry
Sees the individual parts.	Sees the parts as they relate to the whole.
Sees the symptoms a patient has and treats them or refers to another dental specialist for assessment.	See the symptoms a patient has and treats them or refers them to another dental specialist or to holistic practitioners to assess underlying causes that may be coming from physical, mental, or emotional sources.
Gains information from scientific studies to set protocols for care.	Integrates the knowledge gained from anecdotal cases, as well as information gained from scientific studies, to deliver care to each individual.
Works with government agencies in setting regulations for dental care.	Works with a variety of holistic practitioners who assess individuals in an individual way.

An Integrated Look at Dentistry

Here are specific suggestions for integrating holistic concepts into a dental practice. They are derived from my personal experience in a holistic dental office. This model can be applied in teaching the process of care in dental hygiene schools/dental schools as well as for practicing dentists/dental hygienists. The only requirement is to listen and be open-minded.

Amram and Showell, in the introduction to their book, say, "To change your world, *you* must change; *you* must become a new person with a new perspective on life; *you* must dare to pretend" (p. 6). By looking at an example of treatment by the conventional dental hygienist of a patient with recurring gingivitis or gum disease, let us dare to envision what an integrated wellness visit would look like. Let us start by looking at a comparison of the conventional and integrated treatment plans.

The conventional treatment plan

The conventional dental hygienist is trained to perform in the following manner when a patient with gum disease presents for treatment:

- The treatment will be designed to discover symptoms and possible causes, and to suppress symptoms. The mouth is seen in isolation from the body. It is acknowledged, however, that infection can spread to the rest of the body.

- The hygienist will assess the patient's biology and physiology. Some psychological symptoms will be considered, such as stress, when there is attrition or wearing of the teeth.

- The patient's preventive care will consist of cleanings twice a year, or more often if indicated. X-rays will be taken based on the patient's incidence of decay.

- Root planning and scaling is done for patients

with risk factors such as bleeding, tarter below the gums, recession of the gums, or edema.

- Frequency of care and restorations are sometimes based on the amount the patient's insurance will allow.

- Assessments are related primarily to the mouth. Nutrition and habits will be considered.

- Patients are given reasons to change.

- Patients are given suggestions and tracked on a recall system for cleaning and dental exams. The disease's progression is monitored or the patient is referred to conventional practitioners such as medical doctors or dental specialists.

- The practitioner helps make choices for the patient. For example, he or she may recommend cleaning paste containing fluoride, or a rubber dam for restorative work, as well as the materials to be used in restoring the teeth.

- The reassessment of symptoms is done at a recall appointment.

- Options for treatment are backed by protocols and/or scientific research of rational or empirical science. Energy medicine, acupuncture, and traditional Chinese or Tibetan medicines are not acknowledged as options.

- Practitioners recommend solutions to problems. For example, a patient with decay will be given a fluoride treatment in the office or a prescription for at home brush-on fluoride paste, which is stronger than the amount in over-the-counter toothpaste.

- Consultations focus on the mouth and refer to evidence-based scientific studies.

- Follow-ups monitor symptoms, treat symptoms, or point to another approach. When patients have a positive microscopic slide, enzyme test, or toxicity symptoms, changes may be made in home-care techniques, products used, diet, or recall interval. The patient is then referred to the periodontist for treatment of symptoms or to investigate alternatives on her own, without any tracking. The patient decides where to start, without the advantage of assessments of general health status in relation to her dental health and without any support in searching for options that may help her.

Integrated Wellness Plan

The holistic dental practitioner always looks for the cause of disease and how the mouth and teeth are related to and reflect the general health of the patient. The protocol described in the following paragraphs would be used by a holistic dental hygienist after cleaning a patient's teeth, if the hygienist found indicators for periodontal disease. The enzyme test described is available to *all* dental practitioners and is designed to help practitioners obtain objective data that shows there is destruction to the periodontium or the supporting structures of the teeth. This test, called BANA, was described earlier in my discussion of the process of care to show the difference between a conventional and holistic hygienist. I restate some of the BANA process for continuity in explaining the integrated wellness plan and for reader convenience. After a detailed description of this protocol, I will show how the holistic hygienist relates to the patient to discover the cause of the periodontal or gum disease.

The purpose of the BANA (benzoyl-DL-arginine-napthylamide) test is to detect the presence of an enzyme found in three anaerobic bacteria that are associated with periodontitis or destructive gum disease. The test is used to determine if the patient is at risk for future bone loss around the teeth. It is comparable to the use of an x-ray to diagnose caries or cavities. The test results give the dental practitioner a picture of what is happening in the space under the gum tissue. For example, it will tell if there are beneficial bacteria or destructive bacteria present. It is simple to perform and requires only a small sample of plaque placed on an indicator strip that is placed in an incubator for five minutes.

Using the BANA test helps meet the holistic mission and philosophy; the mouth is or can be an expression/ symptom of a deeper cause of an interference in a patient's overall health. It is the holistic dental practitioner's goal to help patients by meeting their dental needs without placing additional stress on their health and to help them discover what the real causes of ill health may be. A positive BANA can be an opportunity for a patient to address the causes of possible ill health and an opportunity for the practitioner to determine if dentistry is a contributing factor.

Another goal is to make patients aware of their risks for future periodontal problems. When they know their risks, they will have the option to act or not act to determine the cause of gum recession.

In a holistic dental office, any adult who wants the

assessment can be tested. The hygienist can evaluate adults eighteen years and older at their recall visits. The dentist can also recommend BANA at any time during treatment or on initial exams. If the patient has *one* of the following indicators, the test would be recommended: recession 1+ mm, pockets 4+ mm, inflammation of the gum, bleeding, abnormal wear of the teeth, or erosion at the gum line of any teeth. The patient then returns for a thirty-minute appointment to conduct the BANA test and discuss the results.

At the BANA appointment, the practitioner tests the areas with the deepest pockets or areas of recession. If the results are negative, the practitioner documents that in the patient's chart. The practitioner discusses options to return for a structural/functional evaluation with the dentist. The goal is to find the cause of the indicator or symptom, namely the recession.

If the results are positive, the practitioner discusses options with the patient. She could return for a wellness consultation to evaluate diet, lifestyle, and medical history or to discuss options for treatment. Or she could take information to another holistic practitioner she already sees for care. The patient can also do nothing.

If the patient chooses to return for a wellness consultation, the practitioner will educate her about holistic philosophy and the mouth as a symptom of deeper health concerns. The practitioner will also take a detailed accounting of the patient's health history from childhood to the present, along with an accounting of diet and lifestyle. The holistic dental practitioner discusses and reviews therapies that the patient has or has not tried, as well as the results. After reviewing the information, the practitioner gives patient suggestions or referrals to conventional and alternative practitioners. In addition, the practitioner discusses follow-up tracking while the patient progresses with alternative care.

The dental hygienist gives the patient the option to arrange follow-up appointments with her to help navigate the holistic care options and to discuss any progress.

At this point, the patient decides whether to participate in the tracking program to discover the underlying causes of the periodontal disease. If she chooses not to participate, the hygienist or dentist could refer her to holistic practitioners to allow her to investigate the condition on their own.

Below is a list of actions for delivering care from a holistic viewpoint during an integrated wellness consultation. This list for an integrated practice is taken primarily from Elliot Dacher's book *Integral Health: The Path to Human Flourishing*. Dacher's concepts for an integrated medical practice have been converted to apply to the approach a holistic dental hygienist would exhibit.

- Practitioner tracks patient as changes are made through a self-discovery program.

- Practitioner makes suggestions and supports the patient as they together make choices in the patient's care. This would include restorative care.

- Assessments include a functional medicine assessment, a lifestyle assessment, and a happiness assessment. Patient will have access to additional assessments for stress and so forth through software on a dental website for sixty days. Practitioner will track patient during the sixty-day assessment period with bimonthly follow-ups.

- Practitioner and the patient explore conventional options as well as holistic alternative options in a partnership-discovery arrangement.

- The practitioner WILL NOT recommend, prescribe, or direct the patient in a search for the underlying cause of symptoms with holistic practitioners (homeopaths, naturopaths, etc.), but rather will support the patient in the discovery of possible options for treatment outside of conventional dentistry.

- The consultation is holistic and patient centered.

- Follow-ups are evolutionary and dynamic.

The components of the integrated wellness consultation are the following: functional-medical assessment tools to determine overall health, lifestyle assessment tools, holistic assessments on traditional Chinese/Tibetan medicine, tracking software, evaluating stages for patients, a process to make changes and discover options for healthcare choices, and follow-up options in tracking progress and promoting positive changes.

The holistic dental practitioner can discuss, perform, or recommend at-home techniques or behaviors to benefit the patient or can refer the patient to other holistic or conventional practitioners for the related factors in the following table:

DENTAL FACTOR	ACTION	REFERRAL/OUTCOME
Acidity in mouth resulting in dental decay	Check with pH strips; discuss diet sugar sources	Nutritionist, naturopath
Attrition/erosion	Discuss effect of grinding/clenching on teeth/bone	Use of night guard or refer to MD, dental TMJ specialist, chiropractic, cranial sacral, or integrated wellness consult
Bacteria, pathological or nonpathological	Irrigation of gum pockets; discuss choices for rinses, toothpastes, or antibiotics	Periodontist, MD, nutritionist, naturopath
Bleeding gums	Discuss possible causes: function, structure, genetics, infection, metabolic imbalance, techniques in home care, chemicals; evaluate home care and technique	Adjust deficiencies in home care and techniques or refer to BANA/microslide; for positive BANA, refer to integrated wellness consult or holistic practitioners
Decalcification/excessive caries (one or more every year)	Evaluate home care and technique, diet; suggest caries-prevention products	Nutritionist and other holistic practitioners
Dehydration/dry mouth	Discuss water intake and quality of beverages; products to promote saliva	MD to check medications
Dental materials toxicity	Discuss option to explore detoxification	Naturopath, traditional Chinese medicine, homeopathy, energy medicine
Excessive plaque, tartar deposits	Homecare techniques and devices	MD, nutritionist, naturopath, or integrated wellness consultation
Environmental toxicity	Discuss option to explore detoxification	Naturopath, traditional Chinese medicine, homeopathy, energy medicine

DENTAL FACTOR	ACTION	REFERRAL/OUTCOME
Lifestyle	Discuss relationship of stress to oral health, stresses on immune system, and deficiency in nutrients	MD, holistic practitioners, integrated wellness consult
Malocclusion or crooked teeth	Functional/structural analysis	Orthodontics
Medical post-op/ radiation	Discuss the effect on oral health; shorten recall, rinses for dry mouth	As indicated to appropriate MD
Mouth breathing, breathing problems, sleep apnea	Discuss effect on oral health and options to protect gum tissue	MD
Nutritional imbalances or deficiencies	Discuss food choices and quality	MD, nutritionist
Overhangs (fillings)	Replacement, restoration, or removal of overhang	Dentist
Recession/pockets	Discuss possible causes: function, structure, genetics, infection, metabolic imbalance, home-care techniques, chemicals to use	BANA appointment; possible referral to periodontist or MD; if positive BANA, then refer to integrated wellness consult or holistic practitioner

In addition to discussing the above dental factors, the practitioner discusses with the patient the following options regarding dental controversies, material choices, dental material compatibility testing, and the retreatment protocols. In this way, patients will become aware of what is available when choosing the dental care they will receive and how that care will be administered.

Dental Controversies

- Patients needing fillings or other restorative work will be given options to test for compatibility to make sure the materials used are not interruptive to the patient's health. They will also be given the option to have metal or nonmetal fillings, whether or not they want amalgam tattoos removed, and which protocol they would prefer upon the removal of the old fillings.

- Root canals or tooth removal, followed by replacement of the missing tooth with a bridge, implant, or partial denture, are options for abscessed teeth. Root-canalled teeth can be filled with different materials and sterilized by different techniques, including lasers.

- Holistic dentists will recommend that all extracted teeth should have the periodontal ligament removed by drilling in order to remove any infection and for bone to regenerate.

- Old extraction sites may have residual infection and result in bone cavitations. The patient will be given the option to have a surgeon retreat these areas with surgery.

- For patients with gum disease, the practitioner will be interested in finding the cause of the disease rather than treating the symptoms with surgery or antibiotics. Root planning and scaling is done only when deposits are present, and not as a general treatment for risk factors such as bleeding and edema.

- Orthodontists vary on whether or not to pull teeth to make room in the patient's jaw when crowding is an issue. Also, patients have the option to have metal brackets or nonmetal. Gold-plated brackets are available and may be less reactive than those containing nickel.

- Holistic dentists will encourage patients with TMJ pain to seek chiropractic, cranial sacral, and other holistic therapies, and to see a dental TMJ specialist.

- Prevention of cavities can be addressed through diet, lifestyle choices, and pH balancing, as well as through an increased use of fluoride.

Dental Material Choices and Compatibility Testing

Holistic-minded practitioners in dentistry and in general are concerned about the materials used to restore the teeth. Metals, when in contact with saliva, generate an electrical current, oral galvanism, releasing mercury vapor, nickel, etc. Furthermore, the nonmetal restorative materials can be interruptive to a patient. Patients can test their sensitivity to materials through blood tests, electrodermal screening, and kinesiology. Sometimes patients use a medical intuitive to determine which materials are most compatible with their body chemistries. These tests are not available in any dental office. Patients will be referred to a lab for blood tests or to other holistic practitioners who do electrodermal screening and kinesiology.

Dental Retreatment Protocols

Holistic dentists often use different protocols when patients request the removal of mercury amalgam fillings or metal crowns to be replaced with another material assumed to be more compatible to the patient's body. This procedure is called retreatment. Hal Huggins's protocol is one of the most well known for retreatment. He recommends the use of blood serum testing with sequential removal of fillings based on electrical reading from the tooth restoration. He uses metals to retreat, while other practitioners recommend no metals be used in dental restorations. Traditional Chinese medicine practitioners see metals in the mouth as contributing to the interference of the body's energy flow. Sources for protocols will be listed in the reference section that follows.

The International Academy of Oral Medicine and Toxicology (IAOMT) recommends that mercury amalgam fillings be removed under cold water spray using copious amounts of water, which the dental assistant vacuums up with high-volume suction. Mercury is released when the removal starts, so patients and practitioners are exposed to the vapor through breathing the fumes. A nasal hood as well as a mask for the dental practitioner is recommended. Air cleaners placed in the treatment room are also recommended. A rubber dam may or may not be used. Practitioners are instructed to wipe the patient's face, replace the paper bib, and replace their gloves after removing the filling material. This will prevent contamination while placing the new filling material. Nutritional and detox information that the patient can put into place before and after treatment can be helpful for the patient undergoing retreatment.

From My Viewpoint

As discussed in Fred Amram's article "Poetry is Dead? So They Say . . . The Future of Labor and the Arts," the scientist will continue to explore, bringing new materials and concepts to help us be more efficient and control our world, while the poet brings meaning to life (Amram, 2008). I see this in my profession of dentistry, in the left-brain, analytical activity of the dentist, and the science we apply. It is right-brain thinking, however, that will help us integrate the concepts that patients need. The personal touch makes the difference in healing. The concepts used in a holistic approach promote health and lead to solutions to solve the problems that patients experience.

The dental profession and patients will benefit from an integrated approach and by recognizing there is an art as well as a science to healing. The art comes from the Eastern concepts of seeing the patient who has the disease rather than seeing the disease the patient has, understanding the body as a complete entity, and recognizing that each individual patient is different. Dentistry can continue to provide us with technology backed by science, but if it is integrated with the knowledge of Eastern philosophy, it will better serve patients. In fact, through the process and approach of an integrated wellness consultation, the dental profession could provide additional benefits it now lacks. When dentistry considers all aspects of conventional and holistic philosophy, it can provide a coherent process of care for dental patients in America.

PART
III

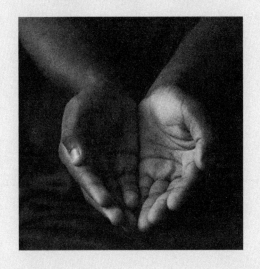

In Your Hands

SIX

How to Take Your Dental Health Into Your Own Hands

Become the change you want to see in the world.

MAHATMA GANDHI

Making Dentistry Whole

The holistic dental professional acknowledges the benefit of conventional dentistry. Patients do, too. If a patient is in pain from an abscessed tooth or a cavity, both patient and practitioner welcome conventional dentistry and its amazing technology. Integration, however, will mean considerable change on the part of the conventional practitioner. Integrating conventional and holistic dentistry means understanding the concepts of holism, accepting there could be a benefit for the patient, educating the dental

83

members in the principles of an integrated dental practice, and then applying the principles in their practices.

The obstacle to integrating is the dominance of left-brain thinking by most dentists. The left brain is rational, mathematical, logical, and scientific. The right brain is more instinctive, intuitive, emotional, spatial, artistic, and creative. The left brain tries to control nature. The right brain is the guide to the inner conscience. Conventional professionals rely on science, rather than feelings, when delivering care to the patient. Yet feelings cannot be destroyed; they must be acknowledged, expressed, accepted, and fulfilled or they will be repressed (Wauters, 1997, p. 131). In order to give coherent care, both the right and left brain need to be acknowledged.

In this chapter, I discuss how dentistry can become integrated by using the principles of coaching; these principles can help practitioners make the changes they need in order to consider all the relevant facts and better serve their dental patient. I also describe how holistic principles can be integrated into the dental school curriculum and what specifically the dentist would be trained to do in order to deliver holistic dental care. Lastly, I recommend that the reader become part of the process of helping the dental profession shift its perspective. By asking questions of the dental professionals who treat them, patients can help their dental caregivers become aware of the need to include holistic concepts and services in their practices.

How to Bring About Change

In their book *Changing for Good*, life coaches James Prochaska, John Norcross, and Carlo DiClemente give a six-step program for overcoming habits in order to make necessary, positive changes. The stages are: the precontemplative stage, the contemplative stage, the preparation stage, the action stage, the maintenance stage, and the recycling stage. A coach recognizes the stages that a person is in by the actions a person does or the words a person uses.

- The **precontemplative stage**: This is the denial phase. It is characterized by statements like "I can't do this" or by a person thinking that something prevents him from making changes. The person may be oblivious and not even know there is a problem.

- **Contemplative stage**: The person knows they need to make changes but may say or imply something like "I don't know how" or "I don't know where to start."

- **Preparation stage**: In this stage, the person has begun to take steps to make changes within thirty days. It is the "I will" phase.

- **Action stage**: This is the "I am" phase. The person carries out changes, preferably with an action plan.

- **Maintenance stage**: This phase involves sustaining the new lifestyle by continually checking on progress to prevent relapse.

- **Recycling stage**: This phase is about learning from any relapses and getting back on track (Prochaska, Norcross, & Diclemente, 1994).

In addition to these stages of change, nine psychological processes are factors in solidifying the changes that one must make to break old habits.

- The first process is **consciousness raising** or making the unconscious conscious. To a dental patient, the practitioner would say, "You have gum disease and it is related to your use of tobacco." This stage is about getting a person's attention.

- **Social liberation** is using the structures already in place by society, if there are any, to help reinforce changes. An example would be smoking bans in public places or the promotion of healthy lifestyles, going green, and so forth.

- The third is **emotional arousal** or **deepening** the feelings about consequences. In order to bring about emotional arousal, a practitioner might say to a patient, "You are more at risk for losing your teeth when you use tobacco, don't floss, have irregular home care, or have infrequent cleanings."

- **Self-reevaluation** is evaluating where a person is now and where she wants to go. A practitioner can help a patient with self-re-evaluation by asking a question like, "How do you feel about smoking? Have you or do you want to quit?"

- **Commitment** is making oneself accountable. This phase includes a person making a private commitment to herself and sharing the commitment in public to increase the chance of success.

- **Countering** substitutes unhealthy behaviors for healthy ones, like enjoyable exercise or participation in another activity that does not connect with the habit.

- **Environmental control** removes temptations from the home/lifestyle or includes the changes. Not having cigarettes in the home or keeping floss in many places as a reminder are examples.

- **Reward** is reinforcement of good new patterns. Often this is left out when changing a negative habit; however, it is extremely important. For every seven days of compliance with the new habit, a person should reward herself with something she desires most. It may be extra time to relax, go shopping, read, or just play.

- **Helping relationships** involve having a support group to help establish a new habit. A person can enlist a friend or family member who is supportive to help her in the process of change (Prochaska et al., 1994).

While it may be easy to see how these stages and processes apply to the elimination of a habit like smoking or the establishment of a habit like flossing, they also can be applied to the integration of holistic concepts into dentistry. The precontemplative stage of change is where many members of the dental profession currently reside. They either think they can't change their ways of doing dentistry or they don't recognize the need to change. These dental professionals are isolated in the profession by being with like-minded individuals, reading like-minded journals, and attending like-minded continuing education seminars. It is uncomfortable for them to integrate anything new into their philosophical frameworks. They are comfortable where they are and are resistant to change.

The dentists in the contemplative stage may acknowledge that some patients have adverse reactions to their dental care, but they don't know how to go about changing. These dentists may make an attempt to get started by using mercury-free materials or doing aesthetic dentistry. They are aware of the danger of dental amalgam and have made a commitment not to expose their staff or patients to it. While they have instituted this policy in their office, they may be unaware of the other controversial subjects in dentistry, or may be unwilling to become totally holistic.

Dentists who are in the contemplative stage have had a consciousness-raising experience at some time. Somehow they became aware of a dental controversy from colleagues or an informed patient who challenged them about why, for example, they still offer amalgam fillings when it has been studied and rejected by the science in other countries.

The following table is a summary of the processes the patient and the dental professional would go through in order to integrate holistic concepts into dentistry.

Process/Stage of Change & Psychological Processes	Patient Centered	Dentist Centered
Precontemplative "I can't" or "I am unaware"	I can't do anything to get holistic care or I don't know it may help me.	I don't know about holistic care or I don't believe it applies to dentistry. There is no scientific evidence.
Contemplative "I don't know how" or "I know I should"	I know my dental work may be affecting my health, but how can I get my dentist to offer it to me?	There are some benefits of holistic practices, but how do I integrate them without endangering my relationship with the American Dental Association?
Preparation "I will"	I will address my concerns with my dentist and ask for holistic techniques. I will prepare educational information for my dentist on holistic techniques so they can be offered to me. I will prepare this for my next visit to the dentist.	I will investigate holistic techniques and integrate them within thirty days. I will address with patients that we have information showing the benefits of these techniques and are integrating them into our practice.
Action "I am"	I have asked for and received holistic care from my dentist.	I offer holistic care to my patients and am open to new techniques within the guidelines of the ADA.
Maintenance "I check" to prevent relapse	I continue to inform myself about holistic care and share that with my dentist.	I continue to update information to offer the best holistic care I can to my patients.
Recycle "I learn" from relapses	I observe my health after dental treatments and note any adverse effects.	I learn new techniques from patients, experiences in conventional dentistry.
Consciousness raising	I share information with my conventional dentist about holistic concepts.	I am open to being confronted by a patient to use holistic techniques and to recognizing that patients have had adverse effects from conventional care.

Process/Stage of Change & Psychological Processes	Patient Centered	Dentist Centered
Social liberation	The Internet offers articles on holism in dentistry.	Holistic concepts are becoming more popular in conventional medicine.
Creating emotion	I project what may happen if I have a root canal, mercury fillings, etc., based on the experiences of other patients who have had adverse effects.	I recognize the growing number of patients who may be affected by conventional dentistry and acknowledge my part in it.
Self-reevaluation	I evaluate the areas in my life where I get holistic care and where I want to go to integrate holistic concepts into my life and healthcare.	I evaluate the holistic services I offer and what else I want to integrate regarding root canals, fluoride, materials testing, etc.
Commitment	I commit to informing my dentist that I want holistic care and to sharing with family and friends.	I commit to informing patients that I integrate holistic techniques into my practice because of my concern for my patients.
Countering	I substitute holistic techniques for nonholistic techniques into my lifestyle and healthcare.	I substitute holistic concepts for conventional in my office.
Environmental	I replace conventional remedies with holistic ones. I replace analgesics with homeopathic remedies.	I replace conventional remedies for holistic ones. I replace analgesics with homeopathic remedies.
Reward	I reward myself for including holistic care into my lifestyle.	I reward myself for including holistic care into my lifestyle and practice.
Helping relationships	I take advantage of the many groups, like the Holistic Dental Association, available for educating myself about holistic dentistry.	I find support from networking with groups like the Holistic Dental Association that help me integrate holistic concepts and techniques.

The most important factor in bringing about change is raising consciousness. This is the first step toward change. My hope is to raise awareness that there is a possibility that American dentistry might be doing harm. In addition, this book could be a blueprint for change to help American dental care to become holistic. By using concepts of systems like traditional Chinese or Tibetan medicine, the dental profession can better serve the public and prevent harm.

My consciousness-raising experience was with a patient and a family member. About ten years ago, Amy called the office of the holistic dentist with whom I worked to inquire about having her mercury fillings removed. A few years earlier, she had had a large amount of dental work done. She had blood tests done that indicated she had very high levels of mercury in her blood. She was twenty-six years old, five feet eleven inches tall, and weighed only ninety-seven pounds. In essence, Amy was dying of mercury poisoning.

The holistic dentist removed her amalgam fillings and within two years she regained her health physically. Emotionally, she had many phobias, one of which prevented her from leaving her home. That is when I worked with Amy as a homeopath to try to help her release her fears homeopathically. It was then that I found out what had exacerbated her body's susceptibility to the effect of the mercury in her dental fillings.

Around the time her fillings were placed, she was the victim of a date rape. She got pregnant and decided to keep the baby. After her daughter was born, she met a man and they decided to marry. The acquaintance rapist then decided to declare his paternal rights and was awarded them by the court. The emotional effects were so devastating that Amy could not detoxify the mercury vapor from the amalgam fillings and the stress on her immune system led to the mercury poisoning. While correlation is not confirmation, the holistic dental practitioner views this experience of trauma as a valid reason her body was unable to detoxify the mercury. And the holistic practitioner says *absence of proof is not proof of absence.*

The mercury poisoning at the core of Amy's story is not a one-time occurrence. Holistic dental professionals believe there are thousands like her. It is an example of the need by the dentist to consider other factors when deciding to place a dental amalgam. The problem, as I see it, is that the ADA has not set up a system for reporting or doing follow-up investigations for cases like Amy's. If there were such a system, member dentists could gain a better understanding of how dentistry can affect individuals in uncharacteristic ways.

My second consciousness-raising experience is personal. In the early 1990s, my husband had a bridge placed from the right lateral incisor to the left central incisor, bridging the gap of the lost right central incisor. He started to have headaches, which worsened over the years. By 2001, he was debilitated, unable to participate in any heavy lifting, and he could no longer participate in golf, his favorite sport. The headaches worsened and the medical doctors, from neurologists to psychiatrists, could not come up with an explanation for the pain. He finally gave up trying to find relief and just endured the discomfort.

One day, he tripped and hit the pavement, knocking out his bridge and his front teeth. A trip to the holistic-minded dentist brought light to the years of headaches he had suffered. The dentist suggested implants or a removable partial, since bridges crossing the midline of the dental arch can lock the palate and cause headaches. The headaches went away never to return. Years of suffering came to an end because a very aware dental professional understood the connection of the mouth to the rest of the body.

These consciousness-raising experiences changed my

life as a dental professional forever. My hope is that the reader may be motivated to ask the question, "How many patients' illnesses are connected to their dental work?" Ignorance of dental controversies like a locked palate is real and changes individual peoples' lives. One knowledgeable dentist can truly help; others unknowingly harm their patients.

Educating Dentists to Be Holistic

Conventional dentists can be taught how to recognize possible cases of dental stress to patients, how to treat them in the office, and how to refer unsuccessful treatment to holistic dentists or holistic practitioners who may offer other helpful treatments. This can be done just as referrals are now made to any other specialty.

When a patient has periodontal pockets, the hygienist will clean and educate the patient on the proper care needed to resolve them. In six months, if the treatment and education is unsuccessful, the hygienist may recommend a shorter recall for cleaning. If this does not work and the pocket worsens, the dentist will refer the patient to a periodontist for treatment. The same procedure can be followed for referring patients to holistic dentists or practitioners when there are unresolved dental complaints or illness.

As mentioned earlier, the key is that the dental practitioner must recognize the connection between the mouth and the body. In the case of gum disease or periodontal disease, the holistic dental practitioner may recognize that the condition relates to home-care techniques, but will also recognize the relationship of the condition to what else is happening in the body. The mouth reflects what is in the body. This reflection may be exacerbated by the patient's dentistry or allergy to metals, or it could be from undiagnosed illness.

What is needed to integrate holism into conventional dentistry is training in holistic concepts. The following is a list of concepts a dentist or auxiliary could be taught with the current conventional approach listed in italics. These concepts are from Elliot Dacher's book *Integrated Health— The Path to Human Flourishing,* with my interpretation of the conventional response to each.

Characteristics of a Holistic Practitioner

- The holistic practitioner considers an individual's biological, worldly, interpersonal, and psycho-spiritual factors. *The conventional approach is to primarily consider only biological factors because the other factors are more subjective.*

- Holistic practitioners acknowledge that changes involve an expansion of knowledge and a transformation. The practitioners expand their knowledge in a horizontal manner and vertically transform themselves, progressing from one step to the next biologically, worldly, interpersonally, and psycho-spiritually. They move from understanding the biological anatomical body to the physiological body to the mind-body and then to the spiritual body. *The conventional approach is horizontal expansion of knowledge based on rational and empirical science. Evolutionary changes are slow. Anecdotal evidence is dismissed. There is no attempt to incorporate the mind and the body.*

- "Holistic" means including all parts of the human experience. *"Conventional" involves a part or parts of the human experience.*

- The holistic philosophy transforms upward in an evolutionary spiral from body to the mind and spirit. *Conventional philosophy primarily includes the body, some psychology, but little spiritual knowledge. Cartesian/Newtonian thought separates the body from the mind and spirit.*

- Holism involves intentional actions rather than *reactive ones.*

- There is a biological spiral that moves from the anatomical body to the physiological body to the mind-body to the spiritual body. *The conventional practitioner primarily sees only the biology and physiology of the person.*

- The worldly spiral moves from survival to creative expression to fulfillment to service. *Survival is emphasized in the conventional approach. Creative expression, fulfillment, and service are desired, but often are rejected for reasons that prevent action. Whether it is fear or closed-mindedness, the conventional approach sticks with objective knowledge rather than ventures into the subjective unknown.*

- The interpersonal spiral moves from me to you to us to all of us. *The conventional approach focuses on you and me.*

- The psycho-spiritual spiral moves from sensory

motor, to the witnessing mind, to calm-abiding, to unity consciousness. *The conventional approach is sensory motor, reacting to emotions and relationships.*

- Knowledge of all preceding approaches is acknowledged and embraced while transcending the limitations of the prior knowledge. *The conventional approach embraces the now and what we know. Conventional practitioners are attached to power and control of their own discipline and they are cautious or suspicious of integrating knowledge outside their own culture. Prior knowledge is often discounted as out of date or inferior.*

- The spiral will involve a new vision, a growth in awareness, and an expansion of ability and skills to treat illness. *The new vision in the mind of a conventional practitioner comes only from more rational scientific studies.*

- An integrated practice includes five guiding principles: holism, evolution, intention, person-centeredness, and dynamism. *A conventional practice controls disease through drugs, surgery, and preventive measures of illness.*

- Practitioners integrate the five principles into their own lives through psychological development and contemplative practice. *Practitioners rely on principles and protocols established by their profession's individual organizations. Protocols and ethics are established based on observations of population masses.*

- Patients are met where they are in their belief systems; trust is built with patience until they are ready to move forward and make changes to promote personal health. *Patients are educated in the accepted principles and knowledge the dental or medical profession accepts.*

- Practitioner and patient are partners in discovering the threads in the patient's story. Deep listening by the practitioner develops a sense of intimacy, empathy, compassion, unity of heart, direct knowledge of the other, an acknowledging presence, and mutual inner peace and stillness as they explore and assess in order to reveal a path for the patient to follow. *Patients are given short amounts of time to explain what is happening. Practitioners are intellectually superior and supply answers for the patient's illness.*

- The diagnosis is an understanding of the cause of the suffering and the obstacles standing in the way, as well as the opportunities for the patient to flourish. *The diagnosis categorizes symptoms into a syndrome with a name, such as periodontal disease, for example.*

- The prescription addresses the inner and outer life of the individual, is tailored to him, and is open to changes and adjustments as needed. *The prescription controls the symptoms.*

- The setting is a place that is physically welcoming and conveys a feeling of sacredness. The practitioner has an open heart and an unconditioned mind. *The office setting may be*

97

cold and clinical and the staff kind but detached,
with a certain belief about what the patient needs.

A conventional practitioner may understand the above characteristics of a holistic practitioner in an integrated practice but may find them overwhelming to even consider implementing. It could take years to learn and to train a staff. Many holistic practitioners have spent years integrating these concepts into their self-understanding and their health practices. While the task might be daunting, I see it as needed and wanted by many health practitioners. Many feel that we must do more than we have been trained to do in institutions of higher learning. These practitioners are frustrated with poor results in resolving some patient complaints.

A study conducted at the Center for Spirituality and Healing at the University of Minnesota entitled "Evaluation of Complementary and Alternative Medicine Rotation in Medical School" revealed that 81 percent of medical students and 88 percent of the medical school faculty believed that CAM (complementary alternative medicine) should be included in the school's curriculum (Torkelson, Harris, & Kreitzer, 2006, p. 30). While we may recognize the need, we need to be realistic about what is necessary to add additional parts to the already-comprehensive curriculum.

Dentistry has long been the beneficiary of wonderful inventions that make the materials we use better, stronger, and more aesthetic. Pain control and patient comfort have improved in my forty years in dentistry. Digital x-rays mean less exposure to radiation. Lasers have changed the way we can treat patients in more effective and painless ways. These inventions have improved dentistry greatly, so what prevents the integration of holistic concepts into the profession?

Where to Find the Answer

I think the answer lies in holistic practitioners seeing their role as involving a movement in stages from survival to creative expression to fulfillment to service. We have been taught to do what we need to survive. We desire creative expression, fulfillment, and service, but often reject them because we deem other things more important. Whether it is fear of losing status as a dental practitioner or just closed-mindedness, the conventional approach is to stick with objective knowledge rather than venture into the unknown and risk rejection by patients or their peers.

To integrate holistic concepts, dental professionals will have to take action and move into a less familiar, more uncomfortable zone. In the book *From Indian Corn to Outer Space*, Fred Amram and Ellen Showell relate the stories of women inventors throughout the history of America. In the early years of this country, women were expected to stay at home and take care of the family. This book shows clearly that many of them went against the grain to come up with the wonderful inventions we use today. We wear pressed clothes, because Mary F. Potts invented the iron. A soldier can wear a vest that is lightweight yet stronger than steel because Stephanie Kwolek invented Kevlar (Amram & Showell, 1995). These women and many others gave us tools to make our lives easier and safer.

Perhaps dental professionals could venture out to give patients more than just better materials, pain control, less radiation, and laser technology. Perhaps they can change the process of care given and recognize the relationship between the teeth and the body. In order to do that, we will have to go against the stream. We will have to challenge our training and the ADA standards, but in so doing, we may discover a way to make dentistry whole. This will mean learning about a philosophy that has simple, basic principles, but is rich with options for treating individual suffering.

Many times, over my many years of study of holistic techniques, I thought I knew it all. Then a patient sat in my chair to reveal yet another holistic therapy I have never heard about. It is humbling to know I will never know it all. The field of holism is so large my arms cannot reach around it. It is comforting to know, however, that I don't have to have all the answers, but only the courage to take another step toward integrating what I know and sharing that with others in my profession who are willing to join me on this journey.

SEVEN

How You Can Help

"You cannot find yourself in someone else.
Of all the people you will meet in a lifetime,
you are the only one you will never leave or lose.
To the question of your life, you are the only answer.
To the problems of your life, you are the only solution."

UNKNOWN

I have examined the potential to integrate the Eastern philosophies of Chinese and Tibetan medicine into conventional dentistry to benefit dental patients. I discussed the practices used by conventional dentists that may be harmful to patients in order to show a need for integration of the holistic model. I also explored the factors that might be preventing the ADA from integrating holistic principles. In addition, I projected what a holistic practice would look like and how integration of Eastern and Western philosophies could be achieved.

101

My greatest wish is to see my colleagues integrate holistic concepts. Reality speaks loudly, however, and I suspect this will never happen in my lifetime. Therefore, I conclude that the patients are the only ones to bring this paradigm shift to the institution of dentistry. The dentists and staff are good people with the best of intentions to help their patients. The patients, I believe, must ask for these changes. The power of the institution will not shift without patients requesting change.

Intimidation Factor

I recently took my son to the emergency room for stitches on a cut too deep for mom to fix. I am always amazed at how small I feel and humbled by a hospital environment. There is the presence of a power bigger than myself that fills me as I walk through the entryway.

We checked in and waited for the triage nurse to check the cut. "When was his last tetanus shot?" she asked. "He was about twelve," I replied. We have declined vaccines for years after my middle son had a seizure shortly after his DPT at age two. The only reason my son had a tetanus shot at age twelve was because my husband took him to the emergency room after he stepped on a nail and wasn't given a choice. That was before cell phones were common and a call to Mom was inconvenient, so he acquiesced to the directive of the professionals.

She lowered her head looking over her glasses and said, "And how old are you now?"

"Twenty-eight," he replied.

"Well, they are going to want to give him a tetanus shot," she said in a firm tone.

"That's fine," I said while my heart started racing. My

mind was prompting me not to back down but to stand for my values. "I want to talk with the nurse first," I mustered.

When the nurse arrived he asked, "You had a question?"

"Yes; can you tell me if the tetanus you have is preserved with mercury?" I asked, watching his body language as I said the words.

He looked puzzled and replied, "I'm not sure."

"Is it in a multidose vial?" I volleyed back.

"I don't really know," he replied.

"If it has mercury in it, we do not want the tetanus," I firmly stated, a bit relieved I was actually able to practice what I preach and not back down.

As a homeopath, I am not opposed to the vaccine, which is based on the law of similars, just as homeopathy is. My objection is to the preservatives used in the multidose vials. Single-dose tubes have no preservatives. I am also concerned about the method of giving vaccines by injection, because this bypasses the natural immune process, although in the case of tetanus the entry is similar: injection or puncture. That said, there are homeopathic remedies to treat tetanus and wounds. I decided not to give the nurse a minilecture about that, however.

This recap of my experience relates the inherent intimidation one feels when encountering the medical profession. Even with all my knowledge and belief in holistic health, I sometimes shutter when taking a stand. But I also know that the kindest thing I can do in those situations is to raise the consciousness of the nurse, in this case to look at the medication he was dispensing and know what he was giving to patients.

This, I believe, needs to happen in dentistry to effectively promote the changes that need to occur to integrate holistic concepts into dentistry. Patients need to ask questions, not to challenge the practitioner, but to inform and raise her consciousness. This can be done with knowledge of holistic concepts and the controversial issues in dentistry discussed in this work and by asking the right questions. The holistic concepts and controversies have been explored in detail earlier in the book. Are you ready for the questions?

What to Ask for When Receiving Dental Care

How will I know if the dentist is holistic? The biggest difference between a holistic dentist and a conventional one is how they see the mouth in relationship to the rest of the body and how they treat what they see.

Conventional dentists acknowledge that an infection in the mouth can cause a problem in the rest of the body. Therefore they will premedicate with an antibiotic if a dental patient has a heart issue like mitral valve prolapse with regurgitation, or if you have had heart surgery or an implant or a transplant. Surgeons treating any of these procedures will discuss the need for premedication with patients when they are to have dental treatment.

In addition to the above, the holistic dentist sees the mouth as a reflection of the body. So when gum recession is present, they suspect a loss of bone throughout the body. This is if they ruled out other factors, such as crooked teeth or the bite. If the tongue has cracks in it, they suspect problems in the patient's digestion. Improper digestion will affect the ability to absorb nutrients necessary to maintain health throughout the body, as well as in the mouth. If there are imprints of the teeth on the tongue, the patient may have dehydration or hypoglycemia. The holistic dentist uses Chinese medicine concepts like tongue diagnostic techniques to determine the mouth-body connection.

Other indicators of a conventional philosophy: Does the dentist place mercury silver fillings, or when placing white composite fillings, does the dentist do materials testing first? Does the office have air filters to remove mercury fumes from the air? Does the practice offer detox information after replacing mercury fillings? Does the practitioner remove the periodontal ligament after extracting a tooth? Does the dentist test for enzymes from pathological bacteria when gum recession is present? Does the dentist refer patients with frequent decay to a nutritionist? Does the practice do nutritional counseling regarding the type of diet for each individual?

Caution . . . If you have answered no to the above questions, the dentist is not holistic. If your dentist rolls his eyes when you ask these questions, he is neither holistic nor open to learning about holistic concepts. This is the most common response I hear from patients requesting holistic care. And the result is that patients may feel the dental professional is unwilling to hear their concerns.

Your questions may be received with a condescending glance or an inquisitive one. The practitioner may be challenged by these questions in two ways. First, she may be upset, feeling that you are challenging her authority, or she may be open to learning more about how she can offer care that benefits their patients.

> **Remember this: your questions may challenge everything they believe in if you have information showing that your dentist is wrong, that suggests your dentist is ignorant about something important, or that will require action on his part.**

Many in the profession are content to practice as they have been taught and not to seek any information that is not from their authoritative source, the American Dental Association.

Therefore, you will need to ask your questions with curiosity rather than with judgment. You might ask, "I am curious; why don't you offer the BANA enzyme test?" rather than "You should offer me the BANA test!" And you can add a little humor to the equation, too. You might say, "After all, you could charge me extra for that test and relieve my mind at the same time. That way we both come out winning!"

A "why" question may carry some judgment, but it is a quick way to cut to the chase. If you sense there is much resistance to your inquiry, you can follow up with, "**What will happen in ten years if we don't know conclusively that I have progressive periodontal disease? Will I be in danger of losing my teeth?**" Asking questions like these will help your dental professional understand that what she decides today may have consequences down the road. It also shows that you are informed and that you will hold her accountable in the future.

In fact, your asking questions could be a conscious-raising experience for your dentist and will likely cause anger or curiosity. Either way, you need to ask questions to promote change. And when you do, the receiving dentist will no longer be in the precontemplative stage. You will have given her enough information to move from the pre-contemplative to the contemplative stage. Your dentist will know that you expect her to inform you about alternatives so you can make informed choices about your dental care.

You are ultimately responsible for your care and are a partner with health professionals, dentists, and medical doctors in making decisions. They need to give you information and options so you can make informed decisions. Conventional dentists do not have the information you have, so you will have to present the information to them.

Together you can then look at the options and choose what you feel is best for you.

When getting your teeth cleaned . . . The purpose of getting your teeth cleaned is to remove hard deposits (tartar) and soft deposits (plaque). These deposits harbor bacteria and have the potential of breaking the ligaments that hold your teeth to the jawbone. The gums may recede and, if left unchecked, can result in tooth loss. You need to know how good your home care is and if you need to do a better job removing the soft deposits by brushing and flossing so that they do not harden when saliva deposits minerals in them. Hard deposits must be removed by a dental professional. Your brushing technique and the frequency of your brushing and flossing can prevent gum disease.

Ask the dental hygienist to use disclosing solution (a red color to detect plaque) at the beginning of your appointment to see if you have been brushing and flossing well enough. Try to brush and floss before you go to your appointment or ask for a brush when you arrive at the appointment. Brush your teeth and floss. The hygienist will be covering your home care with you at some time during the appointment. You will want to know if any bleeding or gum disease issues are from your home-care techniques or may be related to your body chemistry, diet, etc. If you learn at the beginning of the appointment that no plaque is present, you will know that any gum disease present may be from a cause other than your home care. A note of caution: Disclosing solution contains red dye #28. Using it a couple times a year should not be a factor unless you know you are allergic to it.

When you have receding gums . . . Conventional dentistry accepts that patients' gums recede as patients age. When a relatively young person has gum recession, the dentist will often say that the patient brushes too hard. Holistic dentists will assess a cause for receding gums and rarely do they feel it is from brushing too hard. If you have gum recession, you need to know what the factors are and if they may be contributing to gum recession.

Holistic dentists look first at how you bite your teeth together and if you have crooked teeth. If you had braces, there may be some recession if the teeth were moved very far. If you are a diabetic or have osteoporosis or osteopenia, you may be losing the bone around your teeth as the body pulls minerals from the bone to balance the pH of the blood.

Second, the holistic dentist will want to determine if the recession is progressing. Gum recession is very slow and may only recede one, two, or three millimeters over a ten-year period. This doesn't seem like a lot, but over your lifetime, the recession may cause you to lose a tooth.

If you have been told that your gum recession is due to tooth brushing or any other factor, **you may ask for conclusive evidence to see if the recession is progressing by having an enzyme test.** Provide your dentist with the BANA website or ask for a referral to an office that does this procedure. Waiting for ten years to see if recession has progressed does not benefit you.

When having a mercury (silver) filling removed . . . Filling material and even crowns sometimes need to be replaced. The material may crack or a cavity may form around the old filling. It is important for you to know if the tooth has a mercury filling or if a crown has retained mercury underneath it.

As I noted earlier, the International Academy of Oral Medicine and Toxicology (IAOMT) recommends that mercury amalgam fillings be removed under cold water spray using copious amounts of water that the dental assistant vacuums up in the high-volume suction. (Conventional dentists will do this.) Mercury is released from the old filling when the removal starts; patients and practitioners are exposed to the vapor through breathing the fumes. A nasal hood as well as a mask for the dental practitioner is recommended. (The nasal hood is not usually used unless you are getting nitrous oxide. This is not standard in a conventional office.) A rubber dam may or may not be used to prevent scraps of mercury filling from being swallowed. (Some conventional dentists use this to keep the area dry while filling the tooth.)

Practitioners are instructed to wipe the patient's face, replace the paper bib, and replace their gloves after the filling material is removed. This will prevent contamination while placing the new filling material. (This may or may not be done by the conventional dentist.) Nutritional and detox information before and after treatment can be helpful for the patient undergoing retreatment of an old mercury filling. (This is not offered in conventional offices, as they do not acknowledge the risk of mercury contamination by removing an old filling.) **You will need to ask for these precautions when having old fillings removed or crowns replaced. You will need to ask if the crown prep still has mercury filling as part of the tooth. A holistic dentist would remove the mercury and build up the tooth if needed before placing a new crown.**

Holistic dentists remove fillings in a specific order as prescribed by different protocols (e.g., Huggins's protocol). They also measure the electrical activity of the silver filling with a special meter. The results will help them determine in what order to remove the fillings. **You will need to ask for this to be done if you are considering removing more than one of your mercury fillings. You will need to do research about the different protocols used in removing old mercury fillings and then request your dentist follow this procedure.**

Materials testing . . . It is important to consider if the new filling material is compatible with your system when having a filling done or redone.

If your filling is sensitive for weeks after placement, your gum tissue bleeds around a crown without any reason, or Novocain doesn't seem to take during a procedure, it may be that the material is not compatible with you. To make sure you are compatible with the materials your dentist is using, request materials testing. Testing is available through blood tests, electrodermal screening, or kinesiology. **You will need to ask your conventional dentist for this. Say, "I want to be sure the materials you are using to restore my teeth are compatible with my system."** This is important when you are having fillings, crowns, removable dentures, and partials.

Blood tests: Clifford Consulting and Research (www.crlab.com) will test your blood against all the materials used in the dental office and send a report to your dentist identifying the materials with which you are most compatible. You will need to have your blood drawn at a medical facility and have it sent to the Clifford Lab. You do not need to supply the materials being used in the dental procedures. The lab will have them.

Kinesiology or muscle testing: A chiropractor or a naturopath usually performs kinesiology. It is a more subjective test than a blood test and results sometimes vary between practitioners. It is seen as quackery by the medical and dental professions; however, holistic-minded practitioners rely on muscle testing as a tool to identify sensitivities to substances. You will need to supply the materials your dentist intends to use. Holistic offices usually have a kit of all the materials they use available for checkout by the patient.

Electrodermal screening: Chiropractors and many naturopaths use this process to identify sensitivities. It is an objective test using the acupuncture meridians. This test can measure sensitivity to dental materials as well as foods. You will need to bring the materials or kit of materials with you from your dentist.

Caution . . . Your conventional dentist may challenge you to provide evidence showing that these tests are beneficial. Remember that conventional dentistry relies on science that shows what happens most often. In other words, the studies show what happens generally, not individually. They are not concerned with the smaller number of people with reactions to their dental work. The protocols for the profession are based on studies they have chosen to accept.

As covered earlier in this book, they do not accept studies that do not support their philosophy (e.g., studies from other countries on mercury fillings or fluoride). **You will need to be committed to receiving individualized care. Tell your dentist, "I am concerned about what is best for me and I prefer to be tested for sensitivities to the materials you are using to restore my teeth. What harm can it do?"** Remember that the dental profession does not acknowledge the concepts of traditional Chinese and Tibetan medicines. They are content to follow the tradition of science showing what happens most often. But your treatment is about you, the individual. You are unique and require care that fits your body.

When having a tooth pulled . . . Holistic dentists will also remove the periodontal ligament or will request a dental surgeon to remove it.

This procedure will allow the bone to repair without the possibility of healing over infection or remnants of the ligament. Without this procedure, bone may not heal properly, resulting in the formation of a cavitation. This cavity may cause health problems, although I know of no studies confirming this. (That doesn't mean there aren't any. There is plenty of anecdotal evidence.) This is a very controversial topic. I have personally witnessed patients with pain in an extraction site or health problems developing after tooth extraction. Some of them have had retreatment of these areas and indeed infection was found in the sites of extractions done years earlier. **You will need to ask for the periodontal ligament to be removed by drilling, not just by a curette that digs out the ligament, in order to assure its removal.** Surgeons are usually not averse to this procedure, as it makes sense to them. Having a clean wound free from remnants of the ligament will allow for proper healing.

When you have many cavities or decalcified areas . . . Most conventional dentists will recommend a fluoride treatment in patients with an unusual number of cavities or areas of enamel decalcification. Holistic dentists will look for the cause of the frequent decay. They generally do not rely on fluoride treatments, but look for the underlying susceptibility. If there is high sugar use, the holistic practitioner will consider why the patient craves it and what the body needs to be in balance.

Conventional dentists and hygienists have been trained to look for hidden sugars in the diet as a source of frequent decay. The frequency of exposure to these sugars is seen to be the key to frequent decay. Sipping pop all day or chewing gum increases the risk of dental decay. In addition to considering these factors, the holistic dentist looks beyond to the patient's underlying immunity and their susceptibility to decay. What is their diet like, and is it the right diet for them? The conventional dental professional relies on the pyramid diet taught in all the schools as the guideline for good nutrition. The holistic dentist looks to the variety of diets—vegetarian, vegan, metabolic, and combination diet—as a key to understanding the nutritional needs of their patients.

Fluoride is seen as a toxin in the holistic community. This is because of evidence of an increase in hip fractures in areas where the fluoride in the ground water is in parts greater than one part per million. There is also evidence of inhibition of enzymes and dental fluorosis in children. The

American Dental Association no longer recommends fluoride for children ages three and under, although not long ago, fluoride vitamins were given to babies. The question of how much fluoride we get in our drinking water and other substances like toothpaste remains. How much do we need? How much is toxic? Some toothpastes have 1,200 parts per million to more than 20,000 parts per million in the fluoride varnishes popular in dental office treatments today. One part per million in the water supply is considered safe. While you are not eating the products used for the prevention of decay, some is left in the saliva and is available for absorption in the tissues of the mouth.

If you have poor home care (and you will know this because you've asked the dental hygienist before your dental cleaning to show you the amount of plaque you leave on your teeth after brushing) and you have many cavities, better home habits should correct the increase in decay. If you have good home care and still get cavities, then your general immunity may be the culprit.

One question to ask is this: **"Am I on the proper diet to help my immune system protect me against decay?"**

There are a number of possible diets to adopt, and it is important to choose the one suited to you. The pyramid diet is one. This is a one-size-fits-all diet recommended by the Department of Agriculture of the United States Government. It does not consider the needs of the individual person. A vegetarian diet eliminates meat and is popular for ethical and health reasons. The vegan diet further eliminates eggs and dairy products, or other nonhuman animal products. The metabolic diet recommends foods based on how the body metabolizes them. Only a qualified practitioner using information gained from a carbohydrate and protein chase, along with an extensive questionnaire, is able to determine if this is the right diet for you. It is similar to the blood type diet based on an individual's blood type, but is more objective and individualized. The combination diet restricts how foods are to be eaten. For example, it recommends that refined sugars be eaten alone and fruits eaten first. In addition to these, there are many diets that come and go to address different issues, primarily weight loss.

The metabolic diet is popular among those who believe we all need individualized eating plans. This diet, in conjunction with electrodermal screening to determine aversions to different foods, is often used by holistic practitioners. If your dentist is holistic, she will refer you to a holistic-trained nutritionist to assess your individual needs to support your immune system and prevent tooth decay.

The Tibetan and Ayurvedic systems of medicine also have diets for individual types of people. The Tibetan system was described earlier in this book: loong, tripa, and badkan. Different foods help balance these energies.

You will need to ask, **"Who can I go to for an assessment of my diet to see if what I am eating is helping me prevent decay?"**

Your conventional dentist will probably not have anyone to send you to other than a conventional dietitian. You will have to investigate this on your own. You can educate them over time as you seek out these dietary concerns and find sources for help.

When you have pain after a dental treatment . . . It is not uncommon to have pain after dental treatment, especially if you have had Novocain. Holistic dentists often use homeopathic remedies to treat pain.

Homeopathic remedies like *arnica montana* and *hypericum* are used to treat pain after dental treatment. These remedies help the excess fluid from the Novocain injection move away from the injury and help the nerve of the tooth adjust after the trauma of drilling. Consulting with a homeopath is recommended to obtain the right potency for the trauma of the dental treatment. Other natural herbal remedies like calendula tincture or plantain tincture are available to help periodontal pockets heal. Ask your dentist, "**What natural remedies can you suggest that will help the healing or deal with the pain I might have over the next few days?**"

Using *arnica montana* or *hypericum* will stimulate the body to heal or adjust to the injection rather than cover up the symptom by using a pain killer. The conventional dentist may not be able to suggest these, so you will have to research them on your own. You can purchase these remedies over the counter at health food stores in low potency or from a classical homeopath in higher potency. Shopping at a health food store is a good source. Most of them have knowledgeable employees to help you select a natural remedy. Sharing your success with these remedies will help the dentist acquire a positive view of them. Be sure to monitor and record how long it took for symptoms to subside. You can share this with your dentist at your next visit. Holistic dentists like to hear about your healing experience with natural remedies, too.

When a tooth dies or abscesses . . . Conventional dentistry recommends root-canal therapy for a tooth that has died, abscessed, or has deep decay. The holistic dentist informs patients of the risk of root canals, their failure rate, and options for replacing the tooth. The holistic practitioner may recommend trying a natural remedy if it isn't clear that the tooth is dead. (There are tests your dentist can perform that show conclusively if the tooth has died.)

This is a very controversial subject in dentistry. Based on Weston Price's research that I discussed earlier, we know that holistic dentists have grave concerns about root-canal therapy. Root-canal therapy involves embalming a dead tooth, which is then left in the patient's mouth. The risk of further infection is the concern. A tooth has thousands of microscopic miles of tubules in the root that cannot be reached with the embalming fluid. These tubules can harbor infection, according to Price. There is no research I know of that shows otherwise.

Holistic dentists rely on Price's twenty-five years of research to validate their concerns. The failure rate of root-canal therapy is significant in my observation. I do not know of any research that has been done to show the failure rate. But failure can be serious, since it involves an abscess reforming at the root tip or additional pain, even though the tooth is dead. This happens when undiagnosed auxiliary canals are present and not treated or the tooth is cracked.

A dead tooth does need treatment. No homeopathic remedy or herb will remove the infection. I have observed many healers and patients try to do this without success. The infection only expands and bone around the root of the tooth is destroyed. The question is what to do. Holistic thinking says remove the tooth and replace it with an implant or a bridge. The patient ultimately has to weigh the possible risks of the root-canal procedure.

The patient needs to determine the status of the tooth by **asking his dentist if it is dead or if filling the decayed tooth would cause it to die.** And take note: Dentists will do a root canal on a vital tooth if the tooth is in danger of dying because of the trauma of being filled. If the tooth is still alive, homeopathic *hypericum* can be helpful in calming the nerve after the deep decay is removed and filled. In my experience, *hypericum* is a valuable remedy to avert the need for root canals. Holistic dentists commonly use this remedy for nerve/tooth pain.

An existing root-canalled tooth . . . Based on traditional Chinese and Tibetan medicines, the energy meridians run through the teeth. The materials used to restore a tooth or the material used to embalm a root canal will have an effect on other organs that lie on that meridian. The patient could consult a Chinese medicine practitioner to discuss options to counter the negative effects of the root canal. Some alternative filling materials, such Bio-Calex, are less toxic and are available to retreat the canal. **Ask your conventional dentist what material was used to fill the root canal and take that information to your practitioner of Chinese or Tibetan medicine.** Naturopaths and some chiropractors work with detoxification protocols to avert negative effects of dental work as well.

Homeopathic Anecdotes: Success for Trauma and Deep Decay Using Hypericum

Over the years I have heard many stories of healing with homeopathic remedies. Some of the most astounding have been the use of homeopathy in dental treatment. The following stories are from my fellow homeopathic colleagues. They show the importance of integrating alternatives into conventional practices like dentistry.

S. T.'s Story

My son, now twenty-two years old, fell off his bicycle when he was eleven and knocked out his front tooth. The tooth was kept hanging because he was wearing orthodontic braces. I rushed him to the dentist giving him *arnica montana* on the way. She put the tooth back in place and secured it but was doubtful it would survive such excessive trauma. She thought the nerves would be destroyed and asked we return in a few months to take an x-ray to confirm the tooth had died. When we got home I gave him 30c of *hypericum*. It was the only remedy in the repertory for severe nerve damage to teeth. When we returned

117

several months later, she was astonished the tooth was well. At twenty-two, he has beautiful teeth. Hooray for homeopathy!

A. L.'s Story

My son was nine years old when our dentist said he had a horrific cavity in a molar tooth. I was shocked, as this was a permanent tooth, and I couldn't believe he had a cavity! The tooth did not look right, but he had had little sugar in his diet, was breastfed, and never had a bottle. My dentist referred me to a pediatric dentist who wanted to do a root canal. Again, I was shocked. Were there no other options, I questioned? He said the cavity was too deep to fill. The homeopath in me refused to accept this, especially after hearing Dr. King speak about this subject. I contacted my homeopath and asked for a suggestion. She referred me to another pediatric dentist who was more holistic. I was able to get an appointment and the dentist treated my son. My homeopath had armed us with several remedies. The dentist cautioned me the cavity might be too deep to save the tooth, but it was worth a try. The procedure went well and my son had very little discomfort afterward. Today he is eighteen and the tooth is alive. The moral of this story is this: If it doesn't seem right, get second and third opinions. If I hadn't followed my gut, he would have had a root canal for nine years now.

Another Story of a Homeopathic Treatment

My personal story also involves my oldest son. After high school, he was no longer under mother's watchful eye for brushing and flossing. He developed a large cavity in a premolar tooth. It was one that didn't even look like it had decayed from a visual exam, but one look at the x-ray made me gasp! How did this happen? After a consult with Dr. King, he agreed to fill the tooth with the view it might abscess from the trauma of drilling because of how close it was to the nerve. After treatment, I gave him high doses of *hypericum* until the pain resided about one week or so. That was five years ago and the tooth did not abscess. Thankfully, Dr. King and homeopathy came to the rescue.

The Story of Dr. J. M., MD and Homeopath: Tooth Pain Treated with a Constitutional Homeopathic Remedy

My wife came up to me enthusiastically chewing on a piece of pizza. "There is no end to my thankfulness for what you did for me! I can eat and chew without needing to be careful," she said. A few months ago, she saw a dentist for a filling in a wisdom tooth. The filling caused more pain than before it was done. They redid it. The pain worsened. She saw other dentists who could not figure out what was wrong. Eventually, she had the tooth pulled. Contrary to our expectations, it did not resolve the issue. She developed pain in other teeth, even on the other side of her mouth. She could not eat without pain. She had constant pain and became quite irritable because of it. I tried several remedies early in the process but finally gave up, as they did not work. I thought it might be a structural problem with the tooth that would not respond to homeopathy. Given the new developments with the pain traveling around her mouth I decided the problem was not structural. It did not make sense anatomically. Therefore, I looked at the case in a more constitutional manner (the process a homeopath uses to arrive at one remedy to address the whole person, physically, mentally, and emotionally). I really listened to her this time, and not for the description of the pain but to her feelings about the pain and frustration about the "worthless" dentists who caused it! Sometimes it pays to listen to your wife! This time the prescription relieved all the pain of six months in one week. That was a month ago and I am still getting kudos! The point of the story is this: Constitutional treatment often produces the best results and the prescription may not need to be based on physical symptoms alone.

Referrals to Alternative Practitioners

In Dr. Ron King's office, we made a habit of referring patients to alternative healers to help assess and provide answers to dental issues. Some holistic dentists have their own systems to resolve a patient's symptoms. Hal Huggins is a good example. Observing his practice over the years, I've seen him try to balance the body chemistry of patients and saw that he was highly criticized for it. As a result, he lost his license to practice dentistry.

I believe it makes sense to involve other holistic practitioners who are experts in their own field and can bring additional light to search for good health. Referrals to other holistic practitioners protect the dentist with the licensing boards. Informing a patient is usually seen as more educational than diagnostic. We routinely referred patients to the following list of people, although there are probably many more who could be added to the list. The list of alternatives is very rich, I have discovered. The following is a very brief description of alternative healthcare practitioners and why a dental patient may be given the suggestion to consult with them.

Alternative Therapist	What They Offer
HOLISTIC MEDICAL DOCTOR To order medical tests to help in diagnosis and treatment.	They have the benefit of seeing both sides of the coin to guide you in obtaining the best care. A problem is that they are licensed and walk a fine line between conventional medicine and alternative. They have to err on the side of safety to retain their licenses when treating you.
NATUROPATH To integrate alternative therapies, such as those involving herbs, nutrition, and detoxification. They often do electrodermal screening or muscle testing.	Naturopaths are trained to bring your body into balance. They can assess the need to detoxify the system and support it with herbs, nutrition, and homeopathy. Naturopaths have different levels of training and in some cases are licensed. When licensed, they must follow certain protocols to remain licensed. While this process may be seen as protecting the public, it also carries restrictions on the care they offer. You will need to research the area you live in and the individual you work with to get the care you seek. A referral to any holistic practitioner from a trusted source is a good rule of thumb to follow.
Classical HOMEOPATH To prescribe a homeopathic remedy based on the technique used by the founder Samuel Hahneman to stimulate the natural healing response within the client.	Homeopathy is based on the principle of "like helps like." Remedies are chosen based on the totality of symptoms and matched to remedies that have gone through a proving process, exhibiting the same symptoms. Classical homeopaths give one remedy at a time in a variety of potencies based on the vitality of the person. They call this a "constitutional" remedy. They also give remedies for acute situations. An example is *hypericum* for tooth nerve pain. Naturopaths and chiropractors sometimes use homeopathic remedies in this manner. They also prescribe combination homeopathic remedies. Combination homeopathic remedies are easy to find in a variety of stores. Cold-Ez cough drops are an example. These options are viewed by the classical homeopath as addressing the symptom and not the cause of the illness. The classical homeopath rarely recommends a combination remedy, but rather prefers to prescribe one remedy at a time to stimulate the natural, innate healing response of the individual.

Alternative Therapist	What They Offer
CHIROPRACTOR To adjust the spine and musculoskeletal system with nonsurgical procedures.	Chiropractors are considered to be both alternative and mainstream healthcare providers. They can accept health insurance and have greater leeway to integrate alternative methods to relieve patient discomfort. They are licensed, but are not allowed to prescribe drugs for pain. They often recommend nutritional support or herbs and homeopathic remedies. They offer rehabilitative exercises and lifestyle counseling. Some offer adjunct therapies, such as acupuncture, to enhance healing.
ACUPUNCTURE To increase the flow of energy through blocked meridians to promote healing.	This is a part of Chinese medicine. Someone with training performs it. Different levels of training are required by different states. It can be used as an acute treatment or in a constitutional whole-body-balancing manner. Used in Eastern countries for more than 2,500 years for medical treatment.
CHINESE MEDICINE/TIBETAN MEDICINE To assess the cause of discomfort/symptoms. Systems of medicine used for thousands of years.	These closely related systems of medicine involve diagnosing illness by using the client's pulse, tongue, and sometimes urine. Acupuncture and herbs, along with diet recommendations based on body types (Tibetan), help the body overcome illnesses both chronic and acute.
AYURVEDIC MEDICINE To assess and adjust diet and lifestyle to promote health.	This is the Indian system of medicine that balances the patient's system by assessing the body type producing harmony on the physical, mental, and emotional levels with different techniques, including hatha yoga, diet, and meditation.
CRANIAL SACRAL To establish body rhythms by manipulating the bones of the head to create flow in the spinal fluid, in particular resulting in a balance in the form and function of the body.	This therapy is helpful in the body's self-healing and self-regulating ability. A complementary therapy, it is not regulated and education varies among practitioners.
MASSAGE To loosen tight muscles and enhance relaxation.	Helpful in reducing stress in the jaw and throughout the body. Helpful in TMJ complaints from patients.

Alternative Therapist	What They Offer
OSTEOPATH/HORMONE THERAPY To assess hormones levels.	Medical testing assessing the level of all hormones—thyroid, testosterone, progesterone, and estrogen in particular—can be helpful to alleviate dental concerns and overall body health. Particularly helpful in patients with unexplained periodontal disease and early bone loss.
Holistic HEALTH COACH To help patients navigate the alternative maze of options available to obtain the health they seek.	Coaches can help patients identify areas of concern and track them after a wellness consultation, which includes education about holistic philosophy and the mouth as a reflection of the body. Coaches take a detailed health history, from childhood to the present, along with an account of diet and lifestyle. The holistic coach discusses and reviews therapies that the patient has/has not tried, as well as the results. After review of the information, the patient is given suggestions or referrals to conventional and alternative practitioners. In addition, they discuss follow-up tracking while the patient progresses with alternative care. The coach gives the client the option to arrange follow-up appointments with him/her to help navigate the holistic care options and to discuss any progress made. The coaching relationship allows for the client to obtain the goals he/she wants with a system in place to keep on track.

Conclusion

Modern science has in many ways advanced to an extraordinary degree, yet we still persist in a basic form of ignorance which lies at the root of our suffering and results in comprehensive blindness.

PEMA DORJEE, TIBETAN PHYSICIAN (DORJEE, 2005, P. XX)

My long career in dental hygiene has given me years to analyze and observe the work of dentistry. What has surprised me has been my recognition of a simple human fact: To see dentistry through the lens of holism can threaten the conventional practitioner's entire belief system. By agreeing with the principles of Eastern philosophy, conventional dentists would need to make a paradigm shift in how they practice dentistry. It would mean justifying their shift in thinking to their peers, the licensing board, and their patients. This valuable recognition will guide me in interactions with my peers as I move forward to bring the concepts of Chinese and Tibetan medicines into conventional dentistry.

Through the Holistic Lens

Dacher's five principles of healing are valid for me in my daily life. My experience is holistic. I am the full scope of all that is in the human experience, which includes my mind, my body, and my spirit. The world is a part of me and I am a part of the world. Everything I experience is a step-by-step process, beginning with a history of experiences and leading to a shift in consciousness, knowledge, priorities, and capacity. It has been self-generated and self-cultivated. My interpretation of my experiences has been shaped by my perception of what the experiences were. I have for years intentionally and thoughtfully made choices. I recognize that all my experiences are centered in me and I trust that those experiences are meeting my needs. Lastly, I see life as dynamic and ever changing. It is a balancing act of opposite forces striving to maintain harmony and steadiness.

How I See Science

The above concepts affect my philosophy as a dental professional. My focus involves looking at the whole picture and evaluating all the information before drawing conclusions. To my dismay, the profession of dentistry looks at the information and describes it, but doesn't evaluate the effect a protocol or procedure may have on individual dental patient's susceptibility to material sensitivities.

As previously noted, conventional dentistry relies on science to establish practice protocols. But as an x-ray of teeth is a description of things at a moment in time, it is a one-dimensional view of the subject and does not take into

126

consideration all factors. A dental x-ray of the same tooth taken from different angles will show a different perspective of the teeth. Likewise, scientific studies done on the same issue over different time periods or with a different set of researchers can reveal different results.

Scientific studies should be seen as dental x-rays are: They may be a little different in a three-dimensional view and they are not necessarily "the truth." All factors need to be considered. Acknowledging all the variables will help establish a coherent method in standards for dental care.

Holistic therapies must be seen as unique entities and the anecdotal evidence they yield as significant. When integrating these therapies into conventional care, practitioners must understand and consider their strengths and weaknesses in order to bring benefit to patients. Both methods, scientific and anecdotal, have value, and using the information from both will give the dental patient the most benefit.

Because the body is not a machine, I believe it is almost impossible to gain accurate information from science alone to establish protocols in dental healthcare. The body is an interconnected entity of anatomy and physiology, influenced by the mind's perception of the world at any given moment. There are too many variables to predict how a material substance or a procedure will affect any one human body. It is better to observe the individual and understand his/her nature than to predict how an individual will respond to treatment based on the information gained from a scientific study. To me, the reliance on scientific studies alone, when it comes to healthcare, is just not good enough.

Contradiction Diction

By its own admission, the ADA has disposal management plans for dental amalgam. Its refusal to look at all the evidence is at best ignorance of the unique requirements of each individual for good health; at worst, it's stubborn arrogance to admit dentists may be harming the American public. Dental amalgam fillings may have been used for the last 150 years, but that is no longer a reason to continue using them. Dentists should at least be aware that dental amalgam may not be advised for all patients.

In addition, educating dental professionals to suspect mercury poisoning when they see patients with adverse symptoms rather than denying that dental amalgams can hurt the public may be in order. Mercury has been taken out of the paint industry and the medical industry. Maybe the time has come to remove it from the fillings placed in patients' mouths, or at least think about which mouths we are putting it in.

Recommendation 1:
The Need for a Reporting System

Throughout my dental hygiene career, I do not recall any reporting system established by the ADA or state dental board for reporting harm to a patient or any ill effects to a dental patient from dental work. This leads me to question how the ADA can claim that only a small percentage of patients have adverse reactions to conventional dental work. In 1984 the ADA stated in *Science Digest* that only 5 percent of the population was sensitive to dental amalgams and that this statistic was not significant (Huggins,

1993, p. 5). If 5 percent of the American population had any other disease, such as swine flu, it would be considered an epidemic.

I contend that the ADA makes it sound as if the dental work that it endorses is safe. As an organization, it does not respect the needs or unique health considerations of the individual. Hal Huggins's anecdotes, along with the scientific studies of Boyd Haley and other scientists from around the world, suggest that certain dental procedures may harm patients. And without a control measure to report patients with adverse effects, how can the ADA claim that only 5 percent of the population is harmed?

In the foreword to Pema Dorjee's book *The Spiritual Medicine of Tibet: Heal Your Spirit, Heal Yourself*, the Dalai Lama writes, "The difficulty we face in bringing this about [an integrated system of healthcare] is one of communication, for, like other scientific systems, Tibetan medicine must be understood in its own terms, as well as in the context of objective investigation" (Dorjee, 2005, p. xi). A reporting system could establish communication between the conventional dentist and the holistic dentist or holistic healthcare professional. This could become a method for conventional dentists to learn about the connection between dentistry and whole body issues.

Dental professionals already have a reporting system for suspected abuse. Reporting cases of possible harm could easily be facilitated through the public health system or state dental boards and taught in required continuing education classes all dentists go to in order to keep their licensure.

Recommendation 2: More than Mercury

This book is not just about the possible ill effects of dental amalgam. Rather, it is about the ill effects of *all dental procedures and materials* as a whole, and how the integration of another perspective could benefit the dental patient. Dental amalgam was used to demonstrate a concern. My intent is to raise awareness of the possible relationship between a dental procedure and the negative consequences for some people. Conventional dentistry, unlike holistic dentistry, does not acknowledge the patient as an individual. Not all patients have perfectly functioning bodies that can eliminate toxins, for example. When exposed to a dental procedure, one person's body may fail to function properly.

I think dental professionals need to consider this: There is evidence that may not match the science they rely on, and this evidence may show that some patients have been harmed by their dentistry, including the use of amalgam, fluoride, and dental materials in general, as well as by root canals, cavitation, and bridgework. I believe it is time to acknowledge a more inclusive, coherent theory to serve the people with sensitivity (harm) to their dental work. This approach would prevent additional harm to their patients.

Recommendation 3: A Look Within

How would the conventional dentist work with this new philosophy as part of their dental practice? The answer lies in integrating the yin (right brain) of holism with the yang (left brain) of conventional dentistry. This does not entail judging that one is wrong and the other right, but instead advocates the combination of both integrated together.

My hope is to develop concern on the part of the practitioner to question his/her actions in delivering dental care to the patient. Did I place a bridge that may have triggered chronic pain by locking the palate? Does the patient have an allergy to the materials placed, triggering an autoimmune response causing damage to organ systems? Is the chronic pain in an extraction site because of residual pathological bacteria in the jaw? Is the dentistry I deliver today going to exacerbate the chronic illness the patient is experiencing? If the practitioner can honestly face these questions, I hope he/she will search for a way to make sure they are not causing additional harm to the patients.

Summary of Recommendations

- ADA would recognize that a percentage of patients may have adverse reactions to dental procedures.

- The ADA would give dentists permission to study and integrate holistic therapies and holistic knowledge without risk of loss of licensure.

- A reporting system for patients with adverse reactions would be established and anecdotal cases would be published in dental journals to raise awareness.

- Continuing education and certificate programs in complementary alternative medicine (CAM) therapies would be offered to conventional dentists.

- The holistic dentist would be treated like any other dental specialty with a communication system between the conventional dentist, holistic dentists, and other holistic practitioners.

- Conventional dentists develop personal awareness of dental controversies and the mind-body-spirit connection.

- The dental profession needs to remain open to new ideas and other healing systems.

Contented or Complacent

In the final analysis, the most prominent factor preventing integration of traditional Chinese and Tibetan medical concepts into conventional dentistry is the spirit of the dental professional. It is easier to be closed-minded to something one doesn't know than to take a chance and look into a system of effective techniques in another culture. Conventional dentists are content to follow their training of Cartesian/Newtonian science when establishing protocols for practice. They are content to take the observations of science verbatim without seeing the interrelationship of all the parts that make up a human being: the body, the mind, and the spirit.

I am heartened, however, that conventional medicine is making some strides in integrating holistic concepts to benefit patients. An example is that some health insurance companies cover acupuncture and chiropractic treatment. Dentistry could follow medicine to integrate also. Not only do we need a way to acquire and pass information (science), but we need to evaluate all the information from Eastern and Western philosophies to make certain we meet the needs of the patient to prevent illness. And yes, we need to acknowledge that by not integrating these philosophies, dental professionals may be contributing to the chronic illness of some patients.

Carl Jung may be right when he said, "Whatever darkness we are unable to face within ourselves will manifest on the outside . . . this inevitably leads to the projection of our own inner problem onto some other person, group or nation . . . whilst we sit back and proclaim our inner purity and goodness" (Dorjee, 2005, p. 141). I hope that we, as dental professionals, can commit to (1) better serving all the people we treat, and (2) abiding by our pledge in the code of ethics to do no harm. Then, and only then, will dentistry be whole.

If Wishes Were Horses All Beggars Would Ride

My many years in dentistry and observation of the philosophy of dentists tell me the profession will not change without being prompted by the patients they serve. I attended a hearing at the State Board of Dentistry in Minnesota a few years back when Dr. King was on the board. They were addressing the subject of mercury and autism, and several parents of autistic children testified. Advocates for mercury-free dentistry testified also. Then a dentist for the ADA gave testimony, refuting the claim of autism being linked to mercury. He admitted he does not tell his patients there is mercury in the fillings, but rather says that they are "silver fillings." I gasped as I heard his testimony. How could he? What was he protecting that he felt the need to fail to disclose that dental amalgam is 50 percent mercury?

I had hoped Dr. King's eight-year term on the board of dentistry would change things. He had years of experience in holistic dentistry with his own research and anecdotal evidence. His evidence is discounted, just as Weston Price's was almost a century ago. His voice was not heard. Mine will not be heard, either. That is why I reach out to the patients—to the ones who want to prevent possible harm and whose voices haven't been heard, either.

Well-informed patients armed with questions who ask for holistic care while having dental treatment, when heard often enough, will raise the consciousness of the dental profession. Persistence on the part of the patients can only put all of us in a better position to have care based on our individual needs and the health we seek. And perhaps the most important questions of all to the reluctant conventional dentist are these: What could it hurt to try a holistic approach? What do we have to lose? Can we be better off by integrating thousands of years of healthcare knowledge from the ancient systems of Chinese and Tibetan medicines into an organized profession that is only a few hundred years old?

The most important question of all to ask your dentist is this: Are you willing to accept responsibility for not offering me holistic care?

The most important question to ask yourself is: Am I willing to accept responsibility for the consequences for not asking for holistic care and the impact conventional care alone may have on my health?

"Courage is the secret of democracy."

PERICLES

134

Epilogue

The young woman referred to in the preface had a success-
ful kidney transplant. She lives on many medications and
will continue to do so throughout her life. No one will ever
know if the dental bridges containing nickel were the cause
of her kidney failure or exacerbated the lupus.

One thing is certain. If conventional American dentists
practice dentistry for the next 150 years as they have for
the last 150, many more patients may experience the same
misfortune without ever knowing that something as simple as their dental work may be responsible. Unless things
change, the dentists we trust to *do no harm*, may in fact,
be doing just that.

Appendix

Relationship of the Teeth and the Body

Complied from notes of various sources and experiences in holistic dental care and homeopathy.
By Ron King, DDS (2000) and Bette Jo Arnett

Summary of the Tooth: Organ Relationship

Teeth	Organs
upper and lower anterior incisor teeth	bladder and kidney
upper and lower canines	liver and gallbladder
upper right first and second molar	stomach and pancreas
upper left first and second molar	stomach and spleen
lower right and left first and second molar	lung and large intestine
upper right and left premolars	lung and large intestine
lower right premolars	stomach and pancreas
lower left premolars	spleen and stomach
wisdom teeth	heart, small intestine, circulation

PARTIAL LIST OF THE MERIDIAN CHANNELS AS THEY RELATE TO THE TEETH

(Others not included are the muscles, joints, and vertebrae)

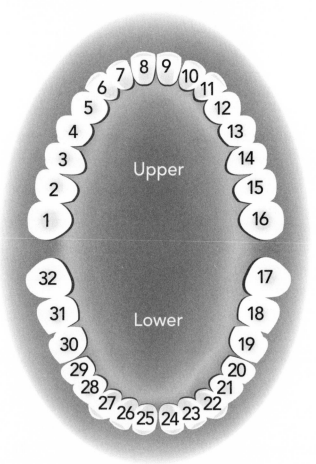

Tooth Number	Sense Organ	Endocrine Gland	Disorders
1, 16, 17, 32: wisdom	1, 16: inner ear 17, 32: ear and eye	1, 16: anterior lobe of pituitary	1, 16: central nervous system, upper extremities, sensory and motor disorders 17, 32: energy, metabolism, peripheral nerves, cervical spine syndromes, blood pressure, sensory and motor disorders See anecdote "Parkinson's disease."
2, 15: upper second molars	maxillary sinus	parathyroid, adrenal, pineal	mammary glands, posterior shoulder pain, arm pain radiating to the ear See anecdote "abscessed tooth" and "breast cancer."
18, 31: lower second molars	ethmoid cells	pineal	inner knee pain, low back pain ascending and descending colon, pelvis and groin issues
3, 14: upper first molars	maxillary sinus	pituitary, thyroid	mammary gland, kidney disorders, vocal cords See anecdote "weight gain."
19, 30: lower first molars	ethmoid cells	pituitary	leg pains, low back pain, sacroiliac joint, hemorrhoids
4, 13: upper second premolars	ethmoid cells, maxillary sinus	thyroid, thymus	digestive issues, gallbladder, liver, valve stenosis, colon
5, 12: upper first premolars	ethmoid cells, maxillary sinus, eye	posterior lobe of the pituitary, thyroid	enzymes, eyes, colon, stomach
20, 29: lower second premolars	maxillary sinus	thyroid	structural issues with hip, knees, feet, mammary glands, lymph
21, 28: lower first premolars	maxillary sinus	gonads	spleen, ovaries, testes, connective tissue and cell respiration
6, 11: Upper canines	eye	posterior lobe of the pituitary	mental emotional disorders from concentration to depression, eye diseases, angina
22, 27: lower canines	eye	gonads	circulation, blood stagnation,
7, 10: upper lateral incisors	frontal sinus	pineal	lymph, immunity, white blood cells count
23, 26: lower lateral incisors	frontal sinus	adrenals	abdominal connective tissue, white blood cell count
8, 9: upper central incisors	frontal sinus	pineal, epididymis	emotional disturbances, from fears to anger and sadness, impotence, hormone imbalances
24, 25: Lower central incisors	frontal sinus	adrenals, epididymis	prostrate, GI tract connective tissue, hormone balances

Anecdotal Experiences

1. **Parkinson's disease:** Male homeopathic client in his early seventies; presented with onset of Parkinson's disease diagnosed two years prior. He had a wisdom tooth pulled a year before the diagnosis of Parkinson's disease. He did not know if the periodontal ligament was removed. The client was unaware of cavitation theory. He chose to see a dental surgeon to retreat the extraction site and remove the periodontal ligament. The surgeon confirmed there was pathology at the old extraction site. The client did report lessening of the Parkinson's disease symptoms over the months following the surgery.

2. **Abscessed tooth:** Homeopathic male client presented with symptoms of pain in left wrist. Client said, "It feels like it is broken." He chose to treat it with chiropractic, acupuncture, and homeopathic remedies with no results over a two-month period. His upper left second molar was bothering him as well and eventually the dentist confirmed it was abscessed. When the tooth was extracted the pain in the wrist resolved over the next few weeks. The left wrist is on the same acupuncture channel as the tooth that abscessed.

3. **Breast cancer:** Female dental patient reported she had been diagnosed with breast cancer in her right breast since her last visit. She wondered if the root canals on the upper molar teeth could be related to the cancer. While this could not be confirmed, it could not be conclusively denied.

4. **Weight gain:** Ten-year-old male client gained excessive weight in the two years prior. Client had a silver filling placed in fourteen, upper left first molar, at age seven. That tooth lies on the same channel as the thyroid. The parents had his thyroid tested and the filling removed. The medical tests showed the thyroid function was within normal limits. No evaluation was done on the pituitary gland. After puberty, additional tests showed estrogen dominance and very low levels of testosterone for a boy his age. Whether or not the teeth and the hormonal imbalance are related could not be confirmed or denied.

PARTS OF THE TOOTH

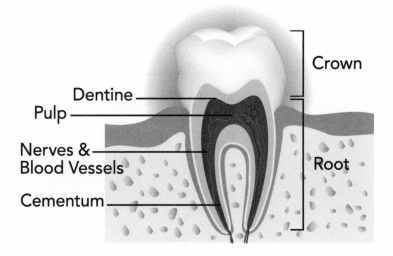

Glossary

abfraction: A worn-away area at the neck of the tooth that may be from a chemical or by trauma during chewing, grinding. or clenching the teeth.

amalgam: The filling material used to restore teeth. Also called "mercury fillings" or "silver fillings" because they contains 43—54 percent mercury and an alloy powder of silver, tin, copper, and sometimes zinc, palladium, or indium.

arnica montana: A homeopathic remedy made from a plant; commonly used by holistic dentists after certain dental treatment (such as extraction or Novocain injections). This helps the body move fluid away from the injury to shorten healing time and reduce pain.

benzoyl-DL-arginine-napthyl-amide (BANA): BANA is a test used to detect enzymes in plaque under gum tissue; the purpose is to determine if pathological bacteria are present. It is used to assess a patient's risk for gum disease. When the enzymes are present the risk is high that gum disease will progress and destroy the tissues surrounding the teeth (ligament, bone, etc.)

bioburden: The accumulation of toxins or bacteria in the body.

chakra: The wheel-like centers or points where energy is filtered through the body. There are seven main chakras. When they are in balance (spinning) they allow energy to flow freely through the system. If they are out of balance (blocked) symptoms of discomfort may appear on the mental, emotional, and physical level. This system is a concept originating in Hindu texts. In Eastern medicine, healing is about bringing the chakras into a balance where all are spinning at the right speed.

complementary and alternative medicine (CAM): The multitude of therapies that can be integrated into conventional care. These include (but are not limited to) acupuncture, homeopathy, massage, hands-on healing, energy work, meditation, traditional Chinese

143

medicine, Tibetan medicine, and Ayurvedic medicine.

conventional care: This term is used to describe the care dentists provide that is in accordance to the guidelines of the American Dental Association and State Boards of Dentistry in each state.

cranial sacral: Bodywork that is gentle and helps resolve physical and emotional issues not helped by other therapies. It helps restore underlying vitality and releases restriction in the body by working on the bones of the skull and the spine to restore the rhythm of the physiological processes of the client.

electro dermal screening (EDS): A method used to assess the vibration of the client in relationship to the vibration of a substance. It is used by a variety of practitioners that are trained in EDS but not necessarily licensed. It is an objective method to assess allergic reactions to substances and is used by holistic dentists to guide them in choosing materials to restore teeth. Dentists refer patients to an EDS practitioner, as using this method is not part of the accepted protocol for dental practices.

erosion: A process of wearing away of the tooth structure, usually by a chemical means. This may be from repeated use of an acid as found in citrus fruits (citric) or in soda pop (phosphoric acid). Additionally,

erosion is seen at the gum line of the teeth and is called an *abfraction*. This may be from repeated trauma to the neck of the tooth as a result of the force of chewing. The weakened enamel then can be eroded by the chemicals in tooth paste or in food.

Focal Infection Theory: The theory that an infection in one area (such as a tooth with a root canal) can affect a person or cause illness in another area of the body.

functional medicine assessment: A medical assessment that reveals how well an individual's body is balanced through an extensive set of questions. The information helps a practitioner focus on areas that need adjustment. Holistic dentists refer patients to other practitioners to conduct this assessment. This assessment can be done by a licensed practitioner, MD, chiropractor, naturopath, or nutritionist.

gum line: The point where the hard structure of the tooth and the soft tissue of the gum meet.

galvanize: The process where an electrical current is created in the mouth because of the presence of two or more metals along with the presence of saliva. The result is the vapor is released into the patient's mouth. Holistic dentists can measure with a machine the amount of electrical current that is released. The dentist will use this information when retreating many teeth to decide the order in which to remove the old fillings.

holistic philosophy: This concept means to treat the whole person—body, mind, and spirit. Holistic practitioners explore and treat the cause of symptoms rather than solely treating symptoms.

holistic practitioner: A person trained in complementary and alternative medicine where by they treat the whole person, taking into consideration mental, emotional, and spiritual aspects of the individual. A conventionally-trained dentist may treat a person holistically without any formal training by referring them to others who offer alternatives like homeopathy, acupuncture, Chinese medicine, etc.

homeopathy: The practice developed in the 1800s by German physician Samuel Hahneman based on the Law of Similars ("Like cures like."). The system uses remedies from three thousand different sources which are diluted to stimulate the natural healing tendency of the human body without toxicity.

hypericum: A homeopathic remedy made from a plant that is specific to nerve injury. Holistic dentists use it after filling a tooth that has deep decay. It may also be used to relive

pain in a tooth that shows no obvious need for treatment. Hypericum helps the nerve of a tooth adjust to trauma either from dental treatment or after outside trauma to a tooth from a fall or blow to the mouth.

integrated wellness plan: This is a proposed outline designed by the author and Ron King to refer dental patients to other alternative medicine practitioners and track them to monitor results or assist them in navigating the many options to resolve their health concerns through holistic means.

kinesiology: A system used by trained holistic practitioners of testing muscles to determine what substances are compatible with a patient's body.

mitral valve prolapse: A condition of the heart where the valve separating the heart's left upper and lower chambers doesn't close properly. A dentist will premedicate a patient with antibiotics to prevent infection when the valve leaks blood from the ventricle into the atrium of the heart (regurgitation).

periodontics: The area that surrounds the tooth and the treating of areas that surround the tooth.

periodonist: A dentist who specializes in treating the gums and restoring the bone around the teeth.

periodontium: The bone and gum tissue covering of the root of the tooth (called the *cementum*) and the ligament that attaches the tooth to the bone.

placebo effect: The measurable effect of a treatment that a patient believes will help them or does help them even though there is no pharmacological substance in it. For example, the client gets better from an infection after taking a sugar pill even though the pill is not an antibiotic.

pocketing: The space caused when a ligament attaching a tooth to the bone is broken.

premedicate: The act of giving a patient an antibiotic before dental treatment to prevent an infection. Commonly used for patients with joint replacements or valve deficiency in the heart

process of care: The process of care is a method used to progress from simple to complex thinking, to critically evaluate what is needed for each individual dental patient. This method is taught in dental hygiene schools and includes assessment, dental hygiene diagnosis, planning, implementation, and evaluation.

recession: Receding of the gums. This can happen because the bone around the teeth is receding.

retreatment: In holistic dentistry, this is the action of removing a filling or bridge to replace it with a material or other treatment that is more compatible with the patient.

rolfing: A form of bodywork that reorganizes the connective tissue or fascia of the client.

rubber dam: This is a piece of rubber that is stretched over a tooth to isolate it from saliva. By keeping the tooth dry it is easier to place the filling material. Holistic dentists use a rubber dam to isolate the tooth when removing the old mercury filling to prevent the mercury filling pieces from being swallowed or the vapor from touching the tissue.

three humours: In Tibetan medicine the individual nature of a person is assessed in terms of *three humours*: Loong, Trip,a and Badkan. These humours represent energy of air, fire, earth, and water, and are always in the body.

toxin: This is a poisonous substance produced within living cells or from a substance that is placed in the body that will produce a toxic effect. An example would be the effect of mercury in dental amalgams.

BIBLIOGRAPHY

ADA. Amalgam. (2010). Retrieved from http://ada.org/prof/resources/topics/amalgam.asp

ADA. Code of Ethics. (2005). Retrieved from http://ada.org/1379.aspx

Aminzadah, K. K. & Etminan, M. (2007). Dental amalgam and multiple sclerosis: A systematic review and meta-analysis. *Journal of Public Health Dentistry*, 67(1), 64-6. Retrieved from http://www.ncbi.nlm.nih.gov/pubmed/17436982

Amram, F. (2008). Poetry is Dead? So they say . . . The Future of Labor and the Arts. *Whistling Shade*. Retrieved from http://www.whistlingshade.com/0801/0801.html

Amram, F. & Showell, E. H. (1995). *From Indian Corn to Outer Space*. Petersborough, PA: Cobblestone Publishing, Inc.

Avey, K. B. (1984). Give your teeth a hug: A simplified brushing technique for children. *Journal of Dentistry for Children*. September–October, 371.

Baum, W. M. (2005). *Understanding Behaviorism: Behavior, Culture, and Evolution*. Malden, ME: Blackwell Publishing.

Baumgartner, J. C., Bakland, L.K., & Sugita, E. I. (2002). Microbiology of endodontics and asepsis in endodontic practice. In *Endodontics*

Bausell, R. Barker. (2007). *Snake Oil Science*. New York, NY: Oxford University Press.

Beinfield, H. & Korngolld, E. (1995). Chinese Traditional Medicine; An Introductory Overview. *Alternative Therapies*. 1(1). Retrieved from http://www.Chinese-Medicine-Works.com/ pdfs/intro_Beinfieldkorngold.pdf

Breiner, M. (2005). Cavitation Treatment. Retrieved from http://www.wholebodydentistry.com

Cameron, M. E. (2001). *Karma and Happiness: A Tibetan Odyssey in Ethics, Spirituality and Healing*. Minneapolis, MN: Fairview Press.

Cameron, M. E. (2004). Ethical Listening as Therapy. *Journal of Professional Nursing*. 20(3), 141–42.

CDC. Community Water Fluoridation. (n.d.). Retrieved from http://www.cdc.gov/fluoridation/other.htm#3

Collis, G. C. (2007). Personal telephone conversation with Bette Jo Arnett.

Dacher, E. (2006). *Integral Health: The Path to Human Flourishing*. Laguna Beach, CA: Basic Health Publications, Inc.

Dodes, J. E. (2001). The amalgam controversy. An evidence-based analysis. *Journal of the American Dental Association*. 132 (3), 348–56. Retrieved from http://www.ncbi.nlm.nih.gov/pubmed/11258092

Dorjee, P. (2005). *The Spiritual Medicine of Tibet: Heal Your Spirit, Heal Yourself*. London, UK: Watkins Publishing.

Frackleton, W., Gastrell Seely, H. (1947). *Sagebrush Dentist*. Pasadena, CA: Trail's End Publishing.

Frawley, D. (2009). *Yoga and Ayurveda, Self-Healing and Self-Realization*. Twin Lakes, WI: Lotus Press.

Geier, D. A., Kern, J. K., & Geier, M. R. (2009). A prospective study of prenatal exposure from maternal dental amalgam and autism severity. *Acta Neurobiolia Experimentalis*. 69(2), 189–97.

Griffin, S. O., Regnier, E., Griffin, P. M., & Huntley, V. (2007). Effectiveness of fluoride in preventing caries in adults. *Journal of Dental Research*. 86(5), 410-415.

Griffith, T. (1997). *Descartes' Key Philosophical Writings*. London, UK: Wordsworth.

Haley, B. (2001). Letter to Dan Burton. Retrieved from http://www.whale.to/m/haley.html

Holistic Dental Association. Our Philosophy (2008). Retrieved from http://www.holisticdental.org

Horowitz, S. (2007). Tibetan Medicine, Ancient Wisdom for Modern Integrative Medicine. *Alternative and Complementary Therapies*. April.

Isham, M. S. (2003). *Ascension! The Analysis of the Art of Ascension as Taught by the Ishayas*. Clemmons, NC: SFA Publications.

Huggins, H. (1993). *It's All in Your Head: The Link between Mercury Amalgams and Illness*. Honesdale, PA: Penguin Putnam, Inc.

Jacobs, J., Jonas, W., Jimenez-Perez, M., & Crothers, D. (2003). Homeopathy for childhood diarrhea: combined results and meta-analysis from three randomized, controlled clinical trials. *Pediatric Infectious Disease Journal*. 22(3), 229-234.

Johnson, H. *Health Coaching Course*. (2008). Retrieved from http://www. healthcoachtraining.com

King, R. (n.d.). Educational Handouts. Retrieved from http://www.kingtooth.com/ handouts.html

King, R. (n.d.). Meridian Tooth Chart. Retrieved from http:// www.kingtooth.com/files/ imtc_secure_king.swf

King, R. (n.d.). Silver Filling Controversy. Retrieved from http://www. kingtooth.com/files/ AMALGAM_5-30-08pdf

Larsen, H. R. (n.d.). Summaries of the latest research concerning amalgam fillings. Retrieved from http:// www.yourhealthbase.com/ amalgams.html

Levy, T. & Huggins, H. (1999). *Uniformed Consent: The Hidden Dangers in Dental Care*. Newburyport, MA: Hampton Roads Publishing.

Levy, T., & Huggins, H. (1996). Cavitation and Extraction Protocol. *Journal of Advancement in Medicine*. 9(4). Retrieved from http://livingnetwor.co.za/ dentalnetwork/cavitation/ cavitation-extrction-protocol/

Mackert, J. R., Jr. (2010). Randomized controlled trial demonstrates that exposure to mercury from dental amalgam does not adversely affect neurological development in children.

Journal of Evidence Based Dental Practice. 10(1), 25–9. Retrieved from http:// www.ncbi.nlm.nih.gov/ pubmed/20230961

Matsuzaka, K., Mabuchi, R., Nagasaka, H., Yoshinari, M., & Inoue, T. (2006). Improvement of eczematous symptoms after the removal of amalgam-like metal in alveolar bone. *Bulletin of Tokyo Dental College*. 47(1), 13–17.

Meinig, G. E. (1998). *Root Canal Cover-Up*. Ojai, CA: Bion Publishing.

Mueller-Joseph, L. & Petersen, M. (1995). *Dental Hygiene Process: Diagnosis and Care Planning*. Albany, NY: Delamar.

Oratec. (n.d.) BANA. Retrieved from http://www.orataec.net/ product

Peterson, G. B. (2004). A Day of Great Illumination: B. F. Skinner's Discovery of Shaping. *Journal of the Experimental Analysis of Behavior*. Nov., 317–28.

Prescrire Int. (2008). No authors listed. Dental Amalgam: few proven harmful affect but many ongoing concerns. *Prescrire International*. 17(98), 246–50.

Prochaska, J. O., Norcross, J. & Diclemente, C. (1994). *Changing for Good*. New York, NY: Harper Collins Publishing.

Radford, B. (2003, January 27). ADA draws criticism—and lawsuits—for stance on amalgams. *The Colorado Springs Gazette*. Retrieved from http://findarticles.com/p/articles/mi_qn4191/is_20030127/ai_n10014923/

Rinpoche, T. W. (2002). *Healing with Form, Energy and Light*. Ithaca, NY: Snow Lion Publication.

Sahakian, W. S. & Sahakian, M. L. (2005). *Ideas of the Great Philosophers*. New York, NY: Harper Collins Publishers.

Shory, N., Mitchell, G. E., & Jamison, H. C. (1987). A study of the effectiveness of two types of toothbrushes for removal of oral accumulations. *JADA Research Reports*. 115-5-717.

Sullivan, K. (2004, May 26). Letter to Minnesota Board of Dentistry. Retrieved from http://www.toxicteeth.org/MinnKipsSummary.pdf

Torkelson, C., Harris, I., & Kreitzer, M. J. (2006). Evaluation of a complementary and alternative medicine rotation in medical school. *Alternative Therapies*. 12, 30–34.

Trabelsi, M., Geurmazi, F., & Zeghal, N. (2001). Effect of fluoride on thyroid function and cerebellar development in mice. *Fluoride*. 34(3), 165–173. Retrieved from http://www.fluoride-journal.com/01-34-3/343-15.pdf

Vithoulkas, G. (1980). *The Science of Homeopathy*. New York, NY: Grove Press.

Wauters, A. (1997). *Chakras and Archetypes: Uniting Energy and Spiritual Awareness*. Berkley, CA: Crossing Press.

Webster, C. (1982). *From Paracelsus to Newton: Magic and the Making of Modern Science*. Cambridge, MA: Cambridge University Press.

Whitworth, L., Kimsey-House, K., Kimsey-House, H., & Sandahl, P. (2007). *Co-Active Coaching: New Skill for Coaching People Toward Success in Work and Life*. Mountain View, CA: Davies-Black Publishing.

Williams, N. J. & Schuman, N. J. (1988). The curved-bristle toothbrush: An aid for the handicapped population. *Journal of Dentistry for Children*. July–August, 291.

Wynbrandt, J. (1998). *The Excruciating History of Dentistry*. New York, NY: St. Martin's Press.